# THE NATURE OF DISEASE

**Philosophical Issues in Science**

Edited by W. H. Newton-Smith

# THE NATURE OF DISEASE

**LAWRIE REZNEK**
BSc, MB, ChB, BPhil, DPhil

ROUTLEDGE & KEGAN PAUL
London and New York

First published in 1987 by
Routledge & Kegan Paul Ltd
11 New Fetter Lane, London EC4P 4EE

Published in the USA by
Routledge & Kegan Paul Inc.
in association with Methuen Inc.
29 West 35th Street, New York, NY 10001

Set in Times
by Witwell Ltd, Liverpool
and printed in Great Britain
by T. J. Press Ltd,
Padstow, Cornwall

Library of Congress Cataloging in Publication Data

Reznek, Lawrie,
The nature of disease.
(Studies in the philosophy of science)
Bibliography: p.
Includes index.
1. Mental illness-Classification. 2. Psychiatric
ethics. 3. Nosology-Philosophy. 4. Medicine-
Philosophy. I Title. II. Series. [DNLM:
1. Disease. 2. Philosophy, Medical. W 61 R434n]
RC455.2.C4 R47   1987    616'.0012    87-9861

British Library CIP Data also available
ISBN 0-7102-1082-5

For my parents
Rose and Koffie
To whom I owe much

# CONTENTS

# ACKNOWLEDGMENTS

Many people have helped with the good ideas in this book, but it would be impossible to name them all. First and foremost I would like to thank Bill Newton-Smith, who read early drafts and made many fruitful suggestions. Jonathan Barnes also read an early draft, providing many insightful comments. Others have helped with individual chapters, and in this connection I would like to thank Simon Blackburn, David Brookes, Jonathan Cohen, Hans Oberdyk, Derek Parfit, Rom Harré, Anthony Quinton, Joseph Raz, Paul and Denise Taylor, and Mark Vincent. I would also like to thank my wife, Eleanor, for her support and for providing a physician's criticism. Finally, according to tradition, I must acknowledge any bad ideas as mine.

I would also like to acknowledge the financial support of the Human Sciences Research Council and the University of Cape Town. Without their help this book would not have been written.

# INTRODUCTION: MEDICINE AND THE NEED FOR PHILOSOPHY

## Why philosophize?

Philosophy is concerned with clarifying our important concepts. It is often accused of being irrelevant. We are told that science teaches us all we need to know about the world, including disease, and that we do not learn anything new from philosophy – it does not enable us to prevent or treat disease.

But philosophy is not irrelevant. It might not help us prevent or treat diseases, but it is relevant to other ends. Concepts carry consequences – classifying things one way rather than another has important implications for the way we behave towards such things. This applies most importantly to the classification of conditions as diseases.

The classification of a condition as a disease carries many important consequences. We inform medical scientists that they should try to discover a cure for the condition. We inform benefactors that they should support such research. We direct medical care towards the condition, making it appropriate to treat the condition by medical means such as drug therapy, surgery, and so on. We inform our courts that it is inappropriate to hold people responsible for the manifestations of the condition. We set up early warning detection services aimed at detecting the condition in its early stages when it is still amenable to successful treatment. We serve notice to health insurance companies and national health services that they are liable to pay for the treatment of such a condition. Classifying a condition as a disease is no idle matter.

This means that clarifying the concept of disease is no idle matter either. If classifying a condition as a disease carries important consequences, then so does the clarification of the exact boundaries of the concept of disease. By deciding that we should draw the boundary of the concept here rather than there, we imply that important consequences obtain with some conditions rather than others. So philosophy is not an irrelevant exercise – science might enable us to decide how to treat the ill, but philosophy enables us to decide whom science should treat.

It might be felt that such a clarification is not necessary, for we all have a grasp of the concept of disease. But a brief survey of medical literature demonstrates that a clarification *is* needed – debates frequently arise over the disease-status of certain conditions. This means that a philosopher has an important role to play.

Let us look at some examples.

## Sickness or poor training?

The paediatrician Noel Preston was asked by the Medical Care Foundation Peer Review Panel whether stuttering was an illness. Insurance companies were refusing to honour claims for its correction because they argued it was not a disease. Their consultants claimed that something was not an illness if it was correctable by education and training, and 'speech therapy is education or training'. One wrote:

> Stuttering is the behavioural manifestation of a group of speech disorders – some of which are clearly neurological, some apparently psychological, and some not yet defined. In the strictest sense, it is the sign of a disorder, not an illness in and of itself (Preston, 1983, p.135).

Noel Preston recommended that the insurance company pay the claim. He argued that something is a disease if it disturbs normal functioning, and that it is not normal to have any difficulty with enunciation and the flow of speech:

> This being the case, stuttering would be a deviation from the normal healthy state. The stutterer is not free from disease or dysfunction, and he does not enjoy all his parts functioning normally. Therefore stuttering is an illness (Preston, 1983, p.135).

This illustrates that debates carrying important consequences arise in the medical domain because the boundaries of the concept of disease need clarification. Far from being irrelevant, the philosopher can make an important contribution to this debate by providing an account of our concept of disease.

## Defect or decay?

Magnavision sold prescription glasses for the condition of presbyopia for a number of years without a licence. The General Optical Council took them to court, arguing that they required to be registered before they could treat defects or diseases. The 1950 Optical Act states that registration with the General Optical Council is required before any agency can treat defects of vision.

Magnavision, on the other hand, argued that presbyopia is not a disease at all. The condition consists in the hardening of the lens of the eye with age, leading to a difficulty with near-vision. They argued that we all suffer from it eventually, and therefore that it is a problem of ageing, and not a disease. Therefore they concluded they did not have to register with the General Optical Council. Here is another issue that can only be settled with a clear understanding of the concept of disease.

## Habit or disease?

A Manchester general practitioner, Dr Chris Steele, prescribed Nicorette, a nicotine-containing chewing gum enabling heavy smokers to give up smoking, for some of his patients. He charged this to the National Health Service (NHS), arguing that the habit of smoking was a disease just like alcoholism, drug addiction, and obesity, and hence that the NHS ought to cover the cost of its treatment as it does for these other addictions.

Such an argument is potentially explosive. If the habit of smoking is classified as a disease, and the NHS required to cover the cost of its medical treatment with Nicorette, it would cost the British taxpayer £20 million a year. In addition, the Treasury could lose hundreds of millions of pounds tax revenue from people who succeeded in giving up smoking! 

The local medical committees supported Dr Steele's view of the matter, but because of the vast sums of money at stake, the Social Services Secretary, Norman Fowler, entered the fray and appealed

3

against this decision. He argued that smoking was not a disease, but rather a bad habit. Just as we do not expect the NHS to pay for the correction of bad table manners, or unsociable habits such as nose-picking, so we should not expect it to pay for the treatment of the habit of smoking!

He went on to claim that patients should pay for Nicorette themselves because it was not a drug. A drug is officially defined as a 'substance that has a pharmacological effect in relation to the prevention or treatment of disease'. His point was that because smoking is just a bad habit, Nicorette is not a drug, and therefore the NHS need not pay for it (as it is not required to pay for caviare or chocolates).

The important issue of whether anti-smoking chewing gum should be charged to the NHS turned on the issue of whether we should classify smoking as a disease, or simply as a bad habit. Here too a philosopher would have been invaluable.

### Symptom or normality?

Throughout the history of medicine there have been extraordinary diagnoses that have received extraordinary treatments. Many normal conditions have been classified as diseases and subjected to horrifying treatments. Such cases illustrate once more that important consequences turn on such a classification, and that there is a need for a clear concept of disease.

In the nineteenth century, masturbation was seen as the symptom of a grave disease. The great English psychiatrist, Henry Maudsley, wrote in 1867 on masturbation:

> The habit of self-abuse notably gives rise to a particular and disagreeable form of insanity, characterized by intense self-feeling and conceit, extreme perversion of feeling and corresponding derangement of thought, in the earlier stages, and later by failure of intelligence, nocturnal hallucinations, and suicidal or homicidal propensities (Maudsley, 1867, p.452).

Once classified as a disease, the medical profession felt justified in subjecting such 'patients' to certain treatments. Alexander Robertson reported that in one American asylum, potassium bromide (a sedative) had become the treatment of choice. This was because the superintendent 'had formerly tried the effect of a silver ring through the prepuce to prevent its retraction, but in their efforts to continue the vile practice it has been torn out' (Robertson, 1869, p.25).

Two English doctors, Bucknill and Tuke, found that potassium bromide was only of temporary value. They tried faradization of the spine, blistering of the prepuce, or a 'constant attendant by day with mechanical constraint by night'. They sadly concluded that no satisfactory means of prevention has yet been devised (Bucknill & Tuke, 1874, p.760).

Dr Spratling considered that to treat masturbation, 'complete section of the dorsal nerves of the penis is a rational procedure but rather too radical for constant routine practice' (Spratling, 1895, p.442). One unfortunate Texan had his penis amputated by a local doctor for the treatment of masturbation (Potts, 1897, 7)!

Similarly, any sexual excess on the part of women was taken to be a sign of a grave illness. Such were the views of female sexuality that the English physician, William Acton, in his treatise *The Functions and Disorders of the Reproductive Organs*, could write:

> I would say that the majority of women (happily for society)
> are not very much troubled with sexual feeling of any kind. ...
> As a general rule, a modest woman seldom desires any sexual
> gratification for herself. She submits to her husband's
> embraces, but principally to gratify him; and were it not for the
> desire for maternity, would far rather be relieved from his
> attentions (Acton, 1857, p.142).

It is hardly surprising with this view of the 'normal' woman that any sexual enjoyment or excess on the part of a woman would be viewed as a symptom of a disease.

Female masturbation was also considered to be a serious illness. Dr Joseph Jones, a leading Louisiana physician, addressed the Louisiana State Medical Society in 1889 thus: 'The excitement incident to the habitual and frequent indulgence of the unnatural practice of masturbation leads to the most serious constitutional effects and in some cases to hopeless insanity.'

Dr Bloch reported proudly in the *New Orleans Medical and Surgical Journal* in 1894 how he had cured a girl of two-and-a-half suffering from resultant 'nervous' symptoms. He excised her clitoris, and was able to report at the time of writing that the child

5

had 'grown stouter, more playful, and had ceased masturbating entirely'.

Similarly, the London surgeon Baker Brown, in the belief that masturbation constituted a grave disease, drew the rational but unfortunate conclusion that it could be cured by clitoridectomy, an operation which he introduced in 1858. A large number of cases were operated upon in his specially instituted London Surgical Home. But he reported that the results were 'by no means satisfactory'!

In 1894, Dr Eyer of the St John's Hospital, Ohio, tried a different method in the treatment of masturbation: he cauterized the clitoris! He also used to fall back on another method of treatment should his first-line therapy fail: a surgeon was called in to bury the clitoris with silver wires – which the child tore out and resumed the habit (Eyer, 1894, p.259).

It took a long while for such views to die down. The 1928 edition of *The Mothercraft Manual* had this to say about children's genital play: 'Untiring zeal on the part of the mother or the nurse is the only cure: it may be necessary to put the legs in splints before putting the child to bed' (quoted in Comfort, 1967, p.113). Similarly, the 1936 edition of Holt's *Diseases of Infancy and Childhood* continued to recommend that masturbation be treated with 'circumcision in boys, and ... circumcision in girls or cauterization of the clitoris' (Holt, 1936, p.154).

Important consequences, then, turned on how female sexuality and masturbation were classified. Classifying a condition as a disease is not an idle matter, and neither is the clarification of the proper boundaries of the concept. Philosophy could not have helped with the 'cure' of such conditions, but it could have prevented such conditions being subjected to such treatments.

It might be objected that although this example shows that important consequences turned on the classification of a condition as a disease, it does not show that we are liable to make the same mistakes now. But this optimism is not justified.

**Disease or way of life?**

The term 'homosexuality' was invented in 1869 by a Hungarian physician, K. Benkert. He wrote:

In addition to the normal sexual urge in man and woman, Nature in her sovereign mood had endowed at birth certain male and female individuals with the homosexual urge, thus placing them in a sexual bondage which renders them physically and psychically incapable – even with the best intention – of normal erection (quoted in Hirschfield, 1936, p.322).

Although there were some dissenters in the medical profession, most doctors agreed that homosexuality was a disease. Edmund Bergler, a Freudian psychoanalytical psychiatrist, argued against such dissenters in his 1956 book, *Homosexuality: Disease or Way of Life?* He classified homosexuality as a neurotic disease, arguing that dissenters neglected the:

fact that *specific* neurotic defences and personality traits that are partly or entirely psychopathic are specifically and exclusively characteristic of homosexuality, and that these defences and traits put the homosexual into a special psychiatric category (Bergler, 1956, p.13).

He was arguing chiefly against the view of Alfred Kinsey, who had produced his first volume, *Sexual Behaviour in the Human Male* in 1948. Kinsey had another explanation for the origin of homosexual behaviour – he believed that it did not arise from any 'neurotic defence mechanism', and hence did not constitute a neurotic disease. He argued that the most important factors in the explanation were:

(1) the basic physiological capacity of every mammal to respond to any sufficient stimulus; (2) the accident which leads an individual into his or her first sexual experience with a person of the same sex; (3) the conditioning effects of such experience; and (4) the indirect but powerful conditioning which the opinions of other persons and social codes may have on an individual's decision to accept or reject this type of sexual contact (Kinsey, 1953, p.447).

There was much at stake in this medical debate. If homosexuals were ill, then the medical profession was justified in subjecting them to various medical treatments. A great deal of time was spent looking for ways in which individuals 'suffering' from homosexuality could successfully be 'cured'. Two psychiatrists describe their treatment:

> A photograph of a male, attractive to the patient, is presented to him and the patient is able to continue to look at this, or remove it as he wishes. If he has not removed it within 8 seconds he receives an electric shock at an intensity previously determined as very unpleasant for him, until he does remove the photograph. The moment he does so the shock ceases. The male stimulus is a signal that something unpleasant is about to happen. Anxiety is evoked by this, and is reduced by avoiding the shock (Feldman and MacCullouch, 1971, p.160).

Far from producing 'healthy' heterosexuals, this method was prone to produce impotent homosexuals!

These methods were not radical enough for some. Dr Fritz Roeder believed that 'homosexuality is a sad pathologic upshot of faulty brain programming'. Believing that this was located in the hypothalamus, he carried out a number of operations on homosexuals, burning out that part of the brain. He reported proudly in the *Medical World News* of 25 September 1970, that this procedure had turned homosexuals into 'tractable human beings'!

Thus debates as to the disease-status of conditions still occur today in spite of our increased knowledge – a philosophic analysis of the concept of disease is still urgently needed.


## Naughty or ill?

There have probably always been restless, fidgety children; children who are too bored with our schools to sit still and pay attention, and who are therefore often disruptive and difficult to manage. In 1934, the paediatricians Dr Kahn and Dr Cohen noted in an article in the *New England Journal of Medicine* that a behavioural syndrome involving short attention span, hyperkinetic behaviour, distractability, and impulsivity, which was a known sequel to encephalitis, could also be observed in children with no known brain damage or illness.

Gradually the idea took hold that such children were suffering from some as yet uncharacterized neurological illness. Maurice

Laufer in 1957 must be credited with 'discovering' the disease of hyperactivity. He wrote:

> It has long been recognized and accepted that a persistent disturbance of behaviour of a characteristic kind may be noted after severe head injuries, epidemic encephalitis, and communicable disease encephalopathies, such as measles, in children. It has often been observed that a behaviour pattern of a similar nature may be found in children who present no clear cut history of any of the classical causes mentioned. This pattern will henceforth be referred to as hyperkinetic impulse disorder (Laufer, 1957, p.38).

Since the 1930s, such children have been treated by the paradoxically sedating stimulant drug methylphenidate (marketed under the trade name 'Ritalin'), becoming drowsy and 'much more manageable'. It has been estimated that up to one million children are presently being sedated by such psychoactive drugs, largely because they are a handful to look after, especially at school (Schrag and Divoky, 1975).

Major consequences turn on the classification of such behaviour as a disease. Without the diagnosis of disease, the pharmacological control of children's behaviour would not have been possible.

## A medical or political problem?

People throughout history have indulged in excessive drinking, and suffered because of it. However, only over the last two centuries has 'habitual drunkenness' been viewed as a disease. It was first classified as a disease by the American psychiatrist, Benjamin Rush, and the English psychiatrist, Thomas Trotter.

Benjamin Rush, in his treatise *An Enquiry into the Effects of Ardent Spirits upon the Body and Mind*, first published in 1785, catalogued the signs and symptoms of the 'disease of inebriety': unusual garrulity and silence, a disposition to quarrel, uncommon good humour and insipid simpering or laughing, profane swearing, rudeness, immodesty, a swollen nose and extravagant acts indicating a 'fit of madness' (Rush, 1785, pp.325-6). Thomas Trotter, in his 1804 *Essay on Drunkenness*, also saw the behaviour of the habitual drunk as a 'disease of the mind'. When the drinker no longer had control over his drinking, then he suffered from this 'disease of the will'.

The medical model was refined by physicians over the two centuries, and culminated in the work of E. M. Jellinek, the Yale psychiatrist and author of the influential work *The Disease Concept of Alcoholism* first published in 1960. He argued that alcoholics differ from people who simply drink excessively in that they have some pathological condition that makes them incapable of exercising control:

> The disease conception of alcohol addiction does not apply to excessive drinking, but solely to the loss of control which occurs in only one group of alcoholics and then only after many years of excessive drinking. The fact that this loss of control does not occur in a large group of excessive drinkers would point toward a predisposing X factor in the addictive alcoholics (Jellinek, 1952, p.674).

The classification of alcoholism as a disease has many consequences, one of which is that alcoholics cannot be found guilty of drunkenness – drunkenness becomes a symptom of the disease of alcoholism. In 1966, Driver, a 59-year-old American who had been convicted more than 200 times for public intoxication, was sentenced to imprisonment for 2 years. Driver appealed, arguing that he was suffering from a disease of the will which led to public drunkenness. The Federal Court of Appeal upheld this defence, and because Driver was classified as ill, he managed to avoid prison (Kittrie, 1971, p.279).

However, within the medical profession over the last few years, there have been objections to the classification of alcoholism as a disease. Robert Kendell, Professor of Psychiatry at the University of Edinburgh, wrote an important article for the *British Medical Journal* in 1970, entitled 'Alcholism: a medical or political problem?' He argues against the classification of alcoholism as a disease:

> The consumption of alcoholic beverages is rising steadily and producing an alarming increase in hospital admissions for alcoholism, convictions for public drunkenness, and deaths from hepatic cirrhosis. The medical treatment of alcoholism is of limited efficacy. There are sound reasons, however, for

believing that all the consequences of alcohol abuse would be reduced if total population consumption could be reduced; and that, within fairly broad limits, total population consumption could be reduced by legislative changes to increase the price or restrict the availability of alcoholic beverages. The conclusion seems inescapable. Until we stop regarding alcoholism as a disease, and therefore as a problem to be dealt with by the medical profession, and accept it as an essentially political problem, for everyone and for our legislators in particular, we shall never tackle the problem effectively (Kendell, 1979, p.370).

This illustrates that debates do arise in medicine as how best to classify conditions, and hence a clear account of the concept of disease would be most useful.

## A role for philosophers

Classifying a condition as a disease is something that carries important consequences, especially for the individual with the condition. Because the classification of a condition as a disease is not an idle matter, so the philosophic clarification of the exact boundaries of the concept of disease is not an idle matter either.

Philosophy cannot cure diseases, but it certainly can cure inappropriate disease-attribution. It can therefore make a real contribution to settling disputes over disease classification, and thereby enable individuals to justly claim medical insurance, to have the treatment of their illness covered by a national health service, to avoid having normal conditions subjected to medical treatment, to avoid being unjustly punished for the symptoms of an illness, and enable us to decide whether the problem should be dealt with by some other institution.

# CHAPTER 1
# INVENTION OR DISCOVERY?

### From anti-psychiatry to anti-medicine

Thomas Szasz is an American psychiatrist who created a revolution in thought with his *The Myth of Mental Illness*. This started a movement that became known as Anti-psychiatry, so-called because he argued that psychiatrists do not discover the diseases they treat, but invent them. He writes:

> When a person does something bad, like shoot the president, it is immediately assumed that he might be mad, madness being thought of as a 'disease' that might somehow 'explain' why he did it. When a person does something good, like discover a cure for a hitherto incurable disease, no similar assumption is made. I submit that no further evidence is needed to show that 'mental illness' is not the name of a biological condition whose nature awaits to be elucidated, but is the name of a concept whose purpose is to obscure the obvious (Szasz, 1973a, p.91).

The obvious is, of course, the procuration of social control of those behaviours (like the shooting of presidents) that we do not like. He writes:

> Psychiatric pioneers invent new diseases and formulate new theories of the etiology of these diseases to justify calling certain preexisting social interventions 'treatments'. Kraepelin invented dementia praecox, and Bleuler invented schizophrenia, to justify calling psychiatric imprisonment 'mental hospital-ization' and regarding it as a form of medical treatment; having new diseases on their hands, they attributed them to as yet undetected defects of the brain (Szasz, 1976, p.38).

Such an important claim – the claim that all psychiatrists are frauds – demands examination. However, in order to claim that mental illness does not exist, Szasz must show that our concept of disease cannot admit such a category. He writes:

> Disease means bodily disease. Gould's Medical Dictionary defines disease as a disturbance of an organ or a part of the *body*. The mind (whatever it is) is not an organ or part of the body. Hence, it cannot be diseased in the same sense as the body can. When we speak of mental illness, then, we speak metaphorically. When metaphor is mistaken for reality and is used for social purposes, then we have the making of myth. The concepts of mental health and mental illness are mythological concepts, used strategically to advance some social interests and to retard others (Szasz, 1973a, p.97).

Thus Szasz argues that because 'patients' with 'mental illness' do not have any underlying physical abnormality, they are not diseased.

The whole anti-psychiatry movement, then, is based on a particular account of the concept of disease. In order to assess the claims of anti-psychiatry, we need to do some philosophy: we need to give a clear account of the concept of disease, and see whether it is indeed necessarily the case that nothing is a disease unless it has an underlying physical abnormality.

But it has not only been psychiatry that has come under fire. Ivan Illich has attacked (physical) medicine itself, arguing that it invents physical diseases too. He believes medicine is guilty of what I will call 'Conceptual Iatrogenesis' – the invention of disease. He claims:

> All disease is a socially created reality. ... In every society the classification of disease – the nosology – mirrors social organization. ... 'Learning disability', 'hyperkinesis', or 'minimal brain dysfunction' explains to parents why the children do not learn, serving as an alibi for school's intolerance or incompetence; high blood pressure serves as an alibi for mounting stress, degenerative disease for degenerating social organization (Illich, 1976, pp.172–4).

The claims of Ivan Illich against physical medicine turn on his claim that medicine invents diseases rather than discovers them. In order to assess the claim, we need to know just what a disease is, and when a disease is genuine. That is, we need to possess a clear account of the concept of disease. In order to assess these charges against medicine and psychiatry, we need to have a philosophic understanding of the concept of disease.

## Values and classification

The history of medicine abounds with examples which seem to show that cultural values influence the way we classify bodily (and mental) conditions. The question arises whether values correctly influence what conditions we classify as diseases, or whether they simply bias our perception of the value-free facts. This question reduces to the question whether the concept of disease is a normative or value-laden notion, or whether it is a purely descriptive or value-free concept. If the concept is a normative one, it ought to express the values of the classifiers, and hence differing cultural values should generate different disease classifications (called nosologies). On the other hand, if the concept of disease is a purely descriptive notion, what conditions are recognized as diseases ought not to be influenced by the values of the classifier.

The debate whether the concept of disease is value-laden I will call the Naturalist–Normativist debate. Normativists are those who believe that the concept of disease is a normative or value-laden notion, and Naturalists are those who believe that the concept of disease is a purely descriptive or value-free notion. One of the aims of this book will be to settle this debate.

Settling this debate has important consequences too. If nosologies simply reflect the values of the classifier, we will not be able to criticize other cultures' classifications for getting things wrong. On this view calling something a disease would be much like calling something a weed. There simply is no value-free fact of weediness that enables us to settle the debate whether Michaelmas daisies are weeds, and so there would be no value-free fact enabling us to settle the debate whether Russian dissidents are ill. Hence, we could not justly criticize Russian psychiatry for making a factual mistake. Whether we can criticize them depends on whether we can show that the concept of disease is not value-laden.

It might seem that our concept of disease is obviously value-laden. This is because many historical examples illustrate that cultural values have influenced the classification of conditions as diseases. The Victorians frowned upon excessive sexual activity. Because of this, excessive seminal loss was viewed as a symptom of the disease which was known as 'spermatorrhoea'. Dr Curling defined this disease in his book *A Practical Treatise on the Diseases of the Testis:*

> The emissions may, however, be more frequent than is consistent with health, and too readily excited, so much so, indeed, as to affect virility, and to give rise to constitutional symptoms of a serious character. These excessive spermatic discharges constitute the complaint termed spermatorrhoea (Curling, 1856, p.386).

The loss could be voluntary, as in intercourse or masturbation, or involuntary as in nocturnal emissions. The French specialist, Dr Lallemand, described spermatorrhoea as a 'disease that degrades man, poisons the happiness of his best days, and ravages society' (Lallemand, 1947, p.ii). No doubt it was the culture's horror of sexuality that made them see spermatorrhoea at the root of many cases of fatigue, parched skin, loss of hair, stammering, deafness, blindness, and so on.

Masturbation was especially abhorred, no doubt also because of the culture's values, and was seen as producing grave long-term physical and psychological sequelae. Henry Maudsley describes the consequences of masturbation begun early in life as follows:

> We have degenerate beings produced who as regards moral character are very much what eunuchs are represented to be – cunning, deceitful, liars, selfish, in fact, morally insane; while their physical and intellectual vigour is further damaged by the exhausting vice (Maudsley, 1868, p.156).

In the same sexually repressive nineteenth century, the childhood expression of any sexual interest was seen as pathological. Dr William Acton invented the disease of 'sexual precocity' in his treatise *The Functions and Disorders of the Reproductive Organs* which first appeared in 1857. He wrote:

> Amongst the earliest disorders that we notice is sexual precocity. In many instances, either from hereditary

predisposition, bad companionship, or other evil influences, sexual feelings become developed at a very early age, and this abnormal excitement is always attended with injurious, often with the most deplorable consequences (Acton, 1857, p.78).

He goes on to recommend 'the shock of cold water falling on the organs' as necessary for the treatment of the condition. Here we see the Victorian values towards sexuality influencing the classification of childhood sexual interest as a disease.

Only until recently was homosexuality *per se* considered a disease. The change in its disease status was brought about by a change in social attitudes – no new fact has been discovered about homosexuality. In the late 1960s Gay Liberation and more militant groups such as the Gay Activists Alliance and the Gay Liberation Front demanded that physicians reclassify the condition of homosexuality. After four years of confrontation, the American Psychiatric Association, influenced by the more tolerant values of the time, voted in 1974 to remove homosexuality *per se* from the class of diseases. Here again we see prevalent social values influencing the classification of a condition as a disease.

In the antebellum southern states of America, black slaves were described as suffering from certain diseases by Dr Samuel Cartwright's 'Report on the diseases and physical peculiarities of the Negro race' published in the *New Orleans Medical and Surgical Journal*, 7 May 1851. He describes the disease 'drapetomania' – 'the disease causing slaves to run away', and 'dysaesthesia aethiopsis' – which caused slaves to 'break, waste and destroy everything they handle – abuse horses and cattle – tear, burn and rend their clothing, and pay no attention to the rights of property'. This illustrates how the values of the white slave-owners influenced their classification of such behaviour. What we would interpret as the healthy protest against an evil system, Dr Samuel Cartwright saw as the manifestation of a disease.

In fact, so influential were these values that the very state of being black was considered to be a disease. Benjamin Rush claimed to have discovered the disease of 'Negritude'. He claimed to have discovered the disease in 1792 when he came across a case of what he took to be a spontaneous cure. Henry Moss was a Negro slave who had depigmented patches on his skin (he was suffering from the disease of vitiligo). Rush took these to indicate a partial spontaneous cure of the disease all Negroes suffered from. This was the disease of Negritude, a mild form of congenital leprosy whose only symptom was the darkness of the skin.

There is a South American tribe most of whose members suffer from the disease of dyschromic spirochaetosis, an infectious disease that carries considerable morbidity and mortality. However, it is characterized by rose-coloured spots on the skin which the tribe find attractive. So much so, that they consider it unhealthy and abnormal to be without the spots, and those who do not have the infection are excluded from marriage (Dubos, 1965, p.54). Again we see that what a culture finds desirable influences the classification of a condition as a disease.

It appears from these examples that a good case can be constructed for the view that the concept of disease is value-laden, and expresses the values (and prejudices) of the culture using the concept. The best explanation, or so it seems, of the fact that the classification of conditions varies with the values of the culture is that the concept of disease is itself a value-laden notion. Just as we might explain why the classification of plants as weeds varies with different people's values by pointing out that the concept of weed is a value-laden notion, so we can explain the variation in disease classification.

Normativists can thus explain why divergent cultural values lead to divergent nosologies. Tristram Engelhardt is a Normativist, and he puts his position thus:

> Disease does not reflect a natural standard or norm, because nature does nothing – nature does not care for excellence, nor is it concerned for the fate of individuals qua individuals. Health, insofar as it is to indicate anything more than the usual functions or abilities of the members of the species, must involve judgments as to what members of that species should be able to do – that is, must involve our esteeming a particular type of function (Engelhardt, 1976, p.266).

That is, the concept of disease is something that reflects our esteeming or positive evaluation of certain states (those that constitute health).

But, it might be argued, if the concept of disease is a normative and not a purely descriptive one, how do we explain the fact that there is such widespread agreement as to what are and are not diseases? We would expect widespread disagreement about what are diseases amongst cultures that do not share the same values. However, what we find is that there is widespread unanimity. People do not disagree with the judgment that TB, or leprosy, or breast cancer are diseases. This is more compatible, it seems, with the view that the concept of disease is a descriptive notion – cultures not sharing the same values but agreeing on the facts would classify the same conditions as diseases if the concept was purely descriptive.

However, the Normativist can argue that the widespread agreement as to the classsification of conditions as diseases testifies not so much to the fact that the concept of disease is descriptive, but rather to the widespread sharing of certain values. As Peter Sedgwick points out:

> Once again, it can be argued that these cultural variations apply only to marginal cases of sickness and health, that there are some physical or mental conditions that are *ipso facto* symptomatic of illness, whether among Bushmen or Brobdig-nagians, duchesses or dockworkers. But there is no reason to believe that the "standardized" varieties of human pathology operate according to a different logic from the "cultural dependent" varieties. The existence of common or even universal illnesses testifies, not to the absence of a normative framework for judging pathology, but to the presence of very widespread norms (Sedgwick, 1973, p.35).

Naturalism, on the other hand, explains why there is such a widespread agreement in a different way. If the concept of disease is a descriptive one, then agreement is reached in spite of the difference in values because the concept does not reflect them. Even Tristram Engelhardt remarks:

> Even if it should be the case that cultural prejudices play a role in judgments that homosexuality or polydactylia are diseases, it would appear that bronchogenic carcinoma and typhoid fever are unambiguously diseases, apart from any reference to particular cultures or ideologies. There appears to be a hard core of disease states the recognition of which as such is not a function of cultural inclinations, much less ideology. Moreover, this hard core seems to be quite broad, including the vast majority of infections and metabolic disease – in fact, all those

diseases with a clear somatic basis which comprise basic human functions (Engelhardt, 1976, p.45).

Christopher Boorse, the leading exponent of Naturalism, puts the view thus:

> Tuberculosis and epilepsy are diseases not because society disvalues them, but because they are cases of biological malfunction. They would not cease to be diseases if some culture developed an admiration for epileptics or consumptives; like anything else, diseases can be assigned a high social status. Within the realm of physiology social judgments of illness are no more infallible than social judgments of the shape of the earth or the number of planets, for they involve claims about the biological constitution of man (Boorse, 1976b, p.89).

How, then, it might be asked, do the Naturalists explain the divergence of disease classification that arises with a divergence in cultural values? Surely this is conclusive evidence that the concept of disease is an evaluative one? But the possibility remains that the concept of disease is a value-free notion, and that cultural values bias cultural beliefs about the value-free facts of the matter.

Values can bias our perception of the facts. For example, many people who disapprove of blacks believe that they are intellectually inferior. The notion of intelligence is defined descriptively in terms of a score on a series of intellectual tasks, and is thereby a descriptive concept. But a person's values can distort his perception of the facts so that he can come to believe that blacks are inferior. It is not that he comes to make one value judgment ('Blacks are intellectually inferior') because he holds another (prejudicial) value judgment. It is that he comes to hold certain beliefs about the fact because of his values.

Similarly, it might be that the concept of disease is a purely descriptive notion, like the concept of an IQ, but that values influence what one comes to call a disease because in this way one's values are supported. For example, it might be that to classify some condition as a disease is to attribute a biological dysfunction. This is a descriptive concept, and one that can be applied independently of one's values. Nevertheless, someone who is prejudiced against homosexuals might *believe* that all homosexuals have a dysfunction because this belief supports and justifies his values. It is nice to believe that the things one condemns are being condemned not just because one dislikes and disvalues them, but because they are *diseases*.

Naturalism is an attractive position because it entails that there is a value-free fact of the matter whether such conditions as smoking or homosexuality are diseases. If the concept of disease is a purely descriptive concept, then we can discover whether some condition is a disease by simply examining the facts, thereby settling cultural disputes. On the other hand, if the concept of disease is an evaluative notion, how do we prevent it being used to enforce the values of those classifying the condition? How can we show that certain classifications are mistaken and certain medical interventions unjustified when any classification expresses the values of the classifier?

When we see that Benjamin Rush classified pigmented skin as a disease, we want to be able to say that he was mistaken. Similarly, when Samuel Cartwright regarded freedom-loving slaves as diseased (with drapetomania), we also want to say that a grave mistake had been made. But if the concept of disease expresses the values of the classifier much like the concept of a weed expresses the values of the gardener, then we cannot say that any mistake has been made – only different values are being held.

In addition, we want to be able to criticize others for making mistakes. For example, we want to condemn Russian psychiatry for including political dissidents amongst those who are suffering from schizophrenia. However, if disease classification is just a matter of expressing values, all we can say is that we have different values. Robert Kendell puts the problem this way:

It would mean that we could never maintain on medical grounds that x or y *were* or were not, diseases. We could only argue on social grounds that they *ought*, or ought not, be *regarded* as diseases. And as the criteria would be social rather than medical such decisions would lie with society as a whole rather than with the medical profession, though doubtless they would be influenced by the effectiveness or otherwise of the treatments medicine had to offer. A further important implication is that we could not criticize Russian psychiatrists for incarcerating sane political dissidents in their beastly asylums: they would be perfectly entitled to regard political dissent as a mental illness if, as is probably the case, most of their fellow-citizens disapproved of political dissenters and it happened to be more convenient to deal with them as patients than as criminals (Kendell, 1975, p.132).

Normativism seems to entail the problem of Relativism. Relativism is the view that the truth of all judgments is relative to one's point of view, and hence that everyone is right (from their own point of view) – in cultural disagreements, no one need be wrong. According to Relativism, drapetmania is a disease from Cartwright's point of view, but not from ours, and there is no absolute point of view in terms of which one is right.

Relativism is an unattractive position. Most of us are not relativists about disease – we feel that Cartwright was wrong absolutely to believe that freedom-loving slaves were diseased, and not simply wrong from our point of view. We feel that Russian psychiatrists are wrong absolutely to classify dissidence as a disease, and not simply wrong from our point of view.

Naturalism, on the other hand, is attractive because it enables us to assume that whether some condition is or is not a disease depends on value-free facts of the matter, and not on the values of the culture. To discover whether smoking or homosexuality is or is not a disease, all we need to do is to examine the facts. That different cultures might value those facts differently should make no difference. And if the disease status of some condition depends on the facts, then we can criticize those who make factual mistakes.

One of the central issues that I will examine in this book is the Naturalist–Normativist debate. As we have seen, a number of consequences turn on the issue of whether the concept of disease is value-laden. If it is value-laden, then we cannot justifiably criticize other nosologies. In addition, medicine appears to take on a repressive face – whatever is found undesirable can be classified as a disease and treated. On the other hand, if the concept of disease is purely descriptive, then there is a fact of the matter as to what are diseases, and medicine cannot be accused of directing itself towards repressing those whom the culture finds undesirable. Rather, medicine is directed towards the cure of 'objective' disease – conditions that can be recognized as such independently of any cultural set of values.

## Inventing diseases

There is another issue I will be examining – the nature of classification. Do we discover the taxonomic (classificatory) divisions that we make, or do we invent them? Do the taxonomic distinctions that we recognize correspond to natural kinds that exist independently of our attempts to classify objects, or do they merely represent convenient ways to code information? There are two separate levels at which this question arises.

The first is at the level of *disease-status*. Here the question is: Is disease-status invented, or do we discover that some condition is a disease? And the second level is that of *disease-identity*. Is disease-identity invented, or do we discover that one condition is the same disease as or a different disease from another condition?

Peter Sedgwick argues that disease-status is invented:

> The blight that strikes at corn or at potatoes is a *human invention*, for if man wished to cultivate parasites (rather than potatoes or corn) there would be no 'blight', but simply the necessary foddering of the parasite-crop. ... Outside the significances that man voluntarily attaches to certain conditions, *there are no illnesses or diseases in nature*. ... The fracture of the septuagenarian's femur has, within the world of nature, no more significance than the snapping of an autumn leaf from its twig: and the invasion of a human organism by cholera-germs carries with it no more the stamp of 'illness' than does the souring of milk by other forms of bacteria (Sedgwick, 1973, p.14).

If Peter Sedgwick is to be claiming anything less trivial than that all our concepts are social creations, he must be claiming that there is no natural boundary dividing conditions that are diseases from those that are not – a natural boundary which exists independently of our nosologies (disease classifications). To make sense of this claim, we will have to examine the idea that there are natural divisions that exist among objects independently of our classifying them.

Not only are there those who see disease-status as something that is invented, there are others who see disease-identity as the product of choices we make, usually based on convenience. Just as the line between disease and non-disease is seen as something we invent rather than discover, so the lines between individual diseases are seen as being invented. On this view, we do not discover that different conditions are the manifestation of a single disease, or that a single condition actually consists of a number of different diseases. Rather, this is something that we decide on the basis of convenience – we 'invent' the distinctions among diseases. As Robert Kendell puts it:

> To our generation it is self-evident that diseases, tuberculosis as well as schizophrenia, are nothing but man made abstractions, inventions justified only by their convenience and liable at any time to be adjusted and discarded. Our present outlook is so whole-heartedly empirical that we find it difficult to credit how an earlier generation could have talked of diseases being 'discovered' like so many golden sovereigns on a beach, or have imagined that there were a finite number of them waiting to be identified (Kendell, 1976, p.24).

Lester King also argues that we do not discover the identity and difference that exists among diseases. Rather, what conditions we take to be manifestations of the same disease (or different diseases) depends on the purpose our classifications serve. He puts the point thus:

> Is puerperal fever a disease entity? Or should we say that the disease entity is the streptococcus infection that happened to localize in the female genital tract and then spread to the peritoneum? Then we note that erisypelas, a distinct clinical entity, is also a streptococcus infection. Even when we make allowances for the differences in bacterial type, should we regard erisypelas and puerperal fever as the same disease entity? We may lump them together if we want, or we may keep them distinct, depending on the purpose that we have in mind. Defining the disease entity is an arbitrary process dependent on context, interest, and usefulness (King, 1984, p.143).

According to this view, then, 'it is wrongly supposed that the classification of diseases is as such a matter of discovery rather than of useful invention' (Margolis, 1976, p.247). The categories of diseases, and of individual disease entities, do not correspond to

24

amazon.com | Johnson's Amazon.com | Books | See all 4 Product Categ

Advanced Search | Browse Subjects | Hot New Releases | Bestsellers |

**Search** Books ▼

*Prime*

You qualify for a FREE trial of Amazon Prime

To get this item by **Monday**

▶ **Buy now and get**

(Lea

SEARCH **INSIDE!**™

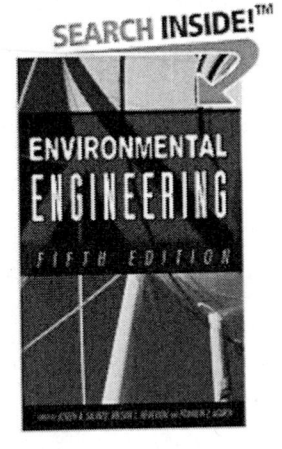

**Environment (Hardcover)**

by Joseph A. Salvat Nemerow (Author), (Author) "Certain ter become familiar are fr communicable and no noncommunicable dis **Key Phrases:** satisfa

Share your own customer images

Search inside this book

any natural divisions or natural kinds that exist independently of our taxonomies.

The theory which holds the taxonomies are neither correct nor incorrect I will refer to as Taxonomic Skepticism (TS for short). Our taxonomies are neither correct nor incorrect because there are no such natural kinds or divisions among objects. In contrast, Taxonomic Realism (TR for short) holds that a taxonomy can be correct or incorrect depending on whether it reflects the natural divisions or natural kinds that exist. If there are such natural divisions, then our taxonomies can be correct (if they mirror these natural divisions) or mistaken (if they fail to correspond to these natural divisions). If such natural divisions exist, then disease-status and disease-identity are things that can be discovered – all we need do is discover where the natural divisions lie.

TR offers the assurance that there is a means of settling the debates as to the disease-status of various conditions, and hence offers an assurance that we will be able to settle how we ought to behave towards the condition. In order to discover whether the NHS should pay for anti-smoking chewing gum, we just need to discover whether smoking falls within the natural kind of disease. In order to discover whether we should put very active children on Ritalin, all we need discover is whether their behaviour falls within the natural division that includes TB and multiple sclerosis. In order to see whether the insurance companies should cover the cost of treating people with stuttering, all we have to do is to discover the natural divisions among bodily conditions. To see whether we are justified in subjecting homosexuals to aversive conditioning, or radical surgery, again all we have to do is to discover what conditions fall into the natural kind of diseases.

The other central theme in this book will be the examination of whether this solution to our classificatory problems is a viable one, or whether the taxonomic divisions that we recognize are invented. We will see whether it is true that if there were no physicians, there would be no diseases. If we discover that diseases constitute a higher order natural kind, then we will have made a case for claiming that disease-status is not something that we invent. If conditions also fall into lower order natural kinds, then a good case can be made for the claim that disease-identity is not something that we invent either.

# CHAPTER 2

# TAXONOMIC REALISM 1: NATURAL KINDS

## Taxonomic realism

There are broadly two opposing views of classification. The first assumes that taxonomies can be correct or incorrect – that is, that there is such a creature as a correct (or mistaken) taxonomy. It supposes that objects in the world are ordered into 'natural' groups or kinds prior to any attempt to classify them, and that it is the job of science to discover such an order (and not to invent it). Classifiers are seen as discoverers, and not inventors.

This is Taxonomic Realism (TR for short). TR is the thesis that taxonomies can be correct or incorrect by either corresponding to or failing to correspond to these natural divisions or kinds. For TR to be correct, two conditions must be satisfied. Firstly, our taxonomic terms must purport to pick out such natural kinds – if they did not, we could not convict the taxonomy of error for not achieving what it did not set out to do. Secondly, the taxonomic terms must actually refer to existing natural kinds.

The second view of classification does not accept that there are such things as natural kinds existing in the world independently of us. Hence there can be no such creatures as correct or incorrect taxonomies – just more or less useful ones relative to different purposes we have for classifications. As there are not natural kinds, taxonomies do not purport to mirror them – they do not pursue truth, but usefulness.

This is Taxonomic Skepticism (TS for short). TS holds that there is no such thing as correct or incorrect taxonomies. There are just more or less useful taxonomies relative to different purposes. For TS to be correct, it must be the case that there are no such things as natural kinds, and our taxonomic terms must not purport to pick them out. Instead, they must simply create groups that are useful.

Let me illustrate the differences between these two views.

Suppose we are wondering whether bats are birds – that is, whether bats fall into the same group as ravens, sparrows, and hawks. According to TR, there is a fact of the matter at stake – we have to discover whether bats fall into the same natural kind that includes other birds. On the other hand, according to TS, the issue is not whether it is correct to classify bats with birds – there is no fact at stake. The issue is whether it is more useful to classify bats with birds, and whether it is more useful depends on the purposes of the classifier. If one is trying to group animals according to the ecological niche that they occupy, it will be more useful to classify bats as birds. However, if one is trying to group animals according to their means of reproduction, it will be more useful to classify bats apart from birds. But neither classification is more correct.

It may be argued that TR is a non-starter – whether bats are birds depends not on any facts in the world, but on what we mean by the words 'bat' and 'bird'. On one definition of 'bird' (something is a bird if and only if it has wings), it is correct to classify bats as birds. On another definition (something is a bird if and only if it has wings and feathers), it is correct to classify bats apart from birds. The correctness of the classification depends not on any facts about natural kinds, but on what we mean by our taxonomic terms. And since meanings are neither correct nor incorrect, no one classification is more correct than another. But if there is no such thing as a (supremely) correct classification, then TR is false. Richard Boyd puts this objection thus:

> According to such a view, it would have been literally nonsense for a seventeenth-century biologist, living in a linguistic community that considered bats to be among the paradigm cases of birds, to claim to have discovered that bats really were not birds, that they lacked the essential features shared by other birds. He could propose to change the meaning of 'bird' to *make it true* that bats did not fall under that term, but there is no such thing as a fundamental principle governing the application of a general term's being mistaken. ... There is simply no such thing as discovering that our fundamental standards of classification are wrong. We can change our standards, of course (by changing the meanings of our terms). It can, perhaps, even be rational to do so – but the rationality cannot be the rationality of correcting a mistaken belief in the face of new evidence (Boyd, 1980, pp.70–2).

27

But this argument is only correct if we assume that our taxonomic terms have a descriptive meaning. If their meaning is given in some other way, the argument would not be valid. Let me illustrate this by using the distinction drawn by the seventeenth-century English empiricist, John Locke, between real and nominal essence.

The nominal essence of some kind, like gold, consists in those observable properties by which that stuff is standardly recognized. The nominal essence of gold consists in a list of properties like being yellow, malleable, shiny, etc. The real essence of gold, on the other hand, consists in the internal constitution of gold which explains why gold has the observable properties it does. This real essence is something that science has to discover, and we know now that the real essence of gold consists in being an atom with 79 protons in its nucleus.

If meanings are descriptive, that is, express nominal essences, then we cannot argue that taxonomies can be correct or incorrect. Whether iron pyrites (sometimes called 'fool's gold' because of its superficial resemblance to gold) are gold depends on how 'gold' is descriptively defined. But once armed with one definition, the question is settled. There is no external standard with which to judge that one descriptive definition is more correct than another.

On the other hand, if terms refer to hidden and as yet unknown real essences, then classificatory mistakes are in principle possible – we can discover we were mistaken to classify iron pyrites as gold when we discover that its real essence is radically different from the real essence of *gold*, and hence it does not belong to the same natural kind. We can correct the boundaries we draw because there is an external standard which we can discover. If our terms purport to pick out real essences, then it is possible for classificatory mistakes to be made. Conversely, as long as our terms express nominal essences, no classificatory mistakes are possible.

So TR is not a non-starter. If our terms purport to pick out natural divisions by referring to real essences, then our taxonomies can be in error when they fail to mirror such natural divisions. Because the natural order is something that we can discover, we can talk of our discovering which taxonomy is correct. On the other hand, if our terms have a descriptive meaning and express nominal essences, we simply invent the distinctions we wish to draw by adopting one definition of our terms rather than another. If we wish to create a division between iron pyrites and gold, we simply define 'gold' in one way rather than another. If we do not wish to, we adopt a different definition. It is up to us.

Let us look at some implications of adopting TR. TR entails that there is a determinate number of kinds existing independently of our taxonomies and awaiting enumeration. If objects fall into natural kinds that we can discover, then it follows that we can discover how many kinds there are by counting the natural kinds we come across. For there to be a determinate number of disease entities, diseases must as a group form a higher-order natural kind, and individual disease entities must on their own form lower-order natural kinds.

To illustrate this, if there were a determinate number of species of fish, animals would have to fall both into the higher-order natural kind of fish as well as into lower-order natural kinds of species. If there was no higher-order natural kind of fish, then whether whales were fish would not be something that we could discover – it would be something we would have to decide by adopting one nominal essence or definition of 'fish' rather than another. If we define 'fish' as 'non-suckling aquatic vertebrate', then there will be $n$ species of fish (where $n$ is the number of species of non-mammalian aquatic vertebrates), but if we define 'fish' as 'aquatic vertebrate', there will be $n+m$ species of fish (where $m$ is the number of species of mammalian aquatic vertebrates). And so how many species of fish we recognize would not be something that was independent of our choice.

Similarly, animals must fall into lower-order (species) natural kinds – if they do not, then whether salmon are regarded as a different species from trout (and not just a subspecies, for example) will not be something that we can discover, but instead something we have to decide. So in order for there to be a determinate number of kinds of fish existing independently of our classificatory system, there must be both higher- and lower-order natural kinds. Similarly for diseases.

In addition, TR entails that one can discover the identities and differences that exist among kinds. And this implies in turn that we discover rather than invent new kinds of things. It is not up to us to decide whether two kinds of things are identical or different – we cannot determine this by adopting one definition of our terms rather than another. Instead, this is something that we have to discover by discovering what natural kinds there are. If we are wondering whether iron pyrites is (a form of) gold, we cannot invent its identity by adopting one definition of 'gold' rather than another. Rather, its identity is something we can and have to discover by seeing whether it falls into the same natural kind or not.

## Medical taxonomic realism

Medical researchers and physicians appear to be Taxonomic Realists – they appear to believe that the identity or difference existing among diseases is something that they have to (and can) discover, that they can discover (rather than invent) new diseases, and that there is a determinate number of diseases existing independently of us.

For example, we find Alois Alzheimer, upon discovering the disease that bears his name, writing:

> We feel that this represents a unique entity. In the last few years more cases have been confirmed. These observations suggest that we should not be content to classify a clinical case without exerting maximal effort to investigate it. There are without doubt many more illnesses than our textbooks describe (Alzheimer, 1977, p.43).

Alzheimer here seems to be adopting TR, for he claims that he has discovered a new disease and he claims that there is a determinate number of diseases existing independently of us. He did not simply claim that it was most convenient to define the condition as being a new disease and not the form of some already known disease, and that it was convenient to think that in the future we could define certain new diseases.

Anton Jacob, in describing the disease now know as Jacob-Creutzfeld disease, wrote in his paper 'Concerning a unique disease of the central nervous system with noteworthy anatomical findings':

> In addition to its clinical individuality, the disease has a very characteristic anatomical substrate. ... I believe I have demonstrated that we have here a unique disease which cannot be denied a nosological niche (Jacob, 1971, p.572).

Jacob argued here that because he had discovered that the nature or real essence of the disease – the 'characteristic anatomical substrate' – was different from any known disease, it was a new disease. He did not claim that he had decided to define the condition as a new disease rather than as the form of some other disease.

In addition, physicians assume that there is a fact of the matter at stake whether some condition is the same disease as another. They do research as if this was something that they could discover. However, if they were Taxonomic Skeptics, this would not be something they would need to discover – it would be something that they could simply decide. For example, there is a debate as to whether the severe neurological disease of infants known as Werdnig–Hoffman's disease is the same disease as the milder neurological disease of juveniles known as Kugelberg–Welander disease.

In 1901, Dr Werdnig described what seemed to be a new disease:

We conclude that we are dealing, in both our cases, with an early infantile, familial muscular atrophy, which resembles dystrophy only in its presentation and in the progressive nature of its development. In the rapidity of its course, however, it bears the distinct signs of a neural illness, and undoubtedly is due to a primary degeneration of the motor pathways of the spinal cord (Werdnig, 1971, p.278).

Somewhat later, in 1956, Drs Kugelberg and Welander thought they had discovered a new and distinct illness:

This type of hereditary juvenile spinal muscular atrophy constitutes a distinct disease entity but seems to be little known, since it is generally mistaken for muscular dystrophy (Kugelberg and Welander, 1956, p.500).

Since then, there has been an ongoing debate as to the identity or difference of these two conditions. Some researchers write:

It is not known at present whether each of these disorders is a separate disease entity (Namba, Aberfeld and Grob, 1970, p.401).

They talk as if the identity or difference of the conditions is a fact of the matter that can be discovered, and not invented. Others write:

31

The question now arises whether Werdnig–Hoffman's disease and the neurogenic infantile muscular atrophies with a slow evolution, are variants of the same disease, or whether they are distinct entities. It does not seem possible to answer this question on the basis of clinical or even anatomical and clinical data, because, a definitive classification is possible only when there is a knowledge of the intimate mechanism causing the abiotrophic diseases in general (Lugaresi, Gambetti and Rossi, 1966, p.404).

Here the physicians seem to argue that there is a fact of the matter at stake as to whether the two conditions are the same disease. They also imply that this is something that we can discover, and discover by uncovering more about the natures or real essences of the conditions (and seeing whether they are identical or distinct). They do not say that their identity or difference is something that will have to be decided upon.

Other physicians also assume that the identity of difference of these diseases is something that we discover, and discover by finding out more about the natures or real essences of the conditions:

Werdnig–Hoffman disease, proximal spinal muscular atrophy of juvenile onset and the adult variants described in the present paper, therefore appear to form a continuous clinical spectrum, and it is questionable whether they represent distinct entities. The varying severities and ages of onset may reflect different degrees of a responsible metabolic defect possibly determined by a gene whose penetration is modified by other genetic and environmental factors. ... On the other hand it is also possible that the metabolic defect may vary from case to case, and the differing patterns of inheritance in the Kugelberg–Welander syndrome provide some support for this. Thus more than one metabolic defect might be capable of disturbing anterior horn function to produce this clinical picture, in the same way that more than one defect may cause other inherited syndrome such as McArdle's syndrome and congenital virilism (Meadows, Marsden and Harriman, 1968, p.548).

This reasoning illustrates again that these physicians think that the identity or difference among diseases is something that is discovered and not invented, and shows they adopt TR. It also illustrates that they think that the fact of the matter is settled by discovering the nature of the disease.

This debate is by no means confined to a single disease. For example, in 1850 Duchenne described the clinical syndrome of Progressive Muscular Atrophy (PMA), a condition leading to progressive wasting of the muscles. In 1874, Charcot described a different clinical syndrome characterized by increasing spasticity which is known as Amyotrophic Lateral Sclerosis (ALS). Although clinically distinct, researchers have argued that the two syndromes represent the same disease because they are due to the same underlying process:

> This review discloses no essential non-clinical [pathological] difference between progressive muscular atrophy and amyotrophic lateral sclerosis. The many similarities in all the investigations can be used to support the view that progressive muscular atrophy is simply a less active or more restricted type of amyotrophic lateral sclerosis (Norris, 1969, p.42)

This is how we would expect physicians to talk if they believed that there was a fact of the matter at stake as to whether the diseases are identical, and if they believed that their identity consists in their having the same real essence.

Thus we can see that debates go on in medicine as to the identity and difference among diseases, and that physicians in the debates appear to believe that the identity or difference is something they can (and have to) discover. They do not believe that these matters are decided by fiat, and hence they appear to embrace TR. Our task now is to see whether TR is correct, and whether the physicians are justified in embracing it.

## Natural kinds

Scientists search for natural classifications of the objects in their domain of study. I must now give sense to the idea that our classifications can reflect a natural order among objects that exists independently of our attempts to classify them. To do this I must give some sense to the notion of a 'natural kind'. William Whewell, a nineteenth-century philosopher of science, thought that when botanists sought for a natural classification of plants, what they were looking for was:

> not of their own creation; not anything merely conventional or systematic; but something which they conceived to exist in the relations of the plants themselves; something which is without the mind, not within; in nature, not in art; in short, a natural order (Whewell, 1840, p.185).

Natural classifications, as opposed to what we might call 'artificial' ones, are thought to reflect an independent order. My task now is to provide some content to this idea. How are we to decide that we have a classification that reflects a natural order rather than some invented order? It is not the case that objects in the world present themselves to us already labelled, so that all we have to do is to read the label to see to what natural kind the object belongs. *We* have to label them, and we must have some means of testing whether our labelling reflects a natural order if the concept of a natural classification is to be given some content. In what follows I will examine some theories as to what natural kinds consist in.

## (1) Whewell's criterion

Suppose we are trying to classify a heap of objects consisting of lumps of different chemicals – emeralds, coal, diamonds, and so on. Let us suppose that we decide to classify them according to size – we classify them into those with a diameter greater than 5 mm, and those with a diameter of less than 5 mm. Is this a natural classification? We feel it is a paradigmatic artificial system because we do not have a logically independent way of drawing the same boundary among these objects. Let us, with Michael Ruse, call this 'Whewell's Criterion' (Ruse, 1973, p.131).

William Whewell argued in his *Philosophy of the Inductive Sciences* that we have a natural classification when 'the arrangement obtained from one set of characters coincides with the arrangement obtained from another set' (Whewell, 1940, p.521). The basic idea is that if the classification does indeed reflect an order that we have not merely invented, then there must be a number of logically independent ways of arriving at the same order. If there is only one way, then it would be unlikely that any natural division among those objects has been reflected. On the other hand, if there were a number of independent ways of drawing the same boundaries among objects, this would be a coincidence that would best be explained if we assumed that there was a natural order independent of us.

However, this criterion is not strong enough, for we *do* have an independent means of drawing the same boundary. We could draw the boundary in the same place if we used the property of having a mass less than $x$ and a density of $a$, or a mass of less than $y$ and a density of $b$, etc. This disjunctive property can draw the boundary in the same place as our property of size, but such a kind is not thereby natural. Such kinds are artificial because there is no reason to draw the boundary here rather than there – drawing it in any one place is arbitrary, and does not coincide with any natural division among the objects. Otherwise we would have to say that the same objects can be classified into infinitely many alternative natural kinds.

## (2) The cluster criterion

On this view, the above kinds are not natural because their members do not have a distinct cluster of properties. A natural kind consists of objects that share a distinct cluster of properties, and we can discover whether our kinds are natural by looking for such clusters. As John Mackie puts its:

> Surely there really are natural kinds, for example chemical elements and compounds (as opposed to mixtures) such as gold, water, common salt, and various species of plants and animals. There are natural kinds because properties are not randomly distributed among things, but tend to cluster. We can say roughly that wherever we find some set of properties – those that could be used as a defining set for, say cats – we also find many other properties common to the class of objects picked out by the first set, including a number of other sets of properties each of which would serve as an alternative defining set for that class, being distinctive of, as well as common to, cats. Admittedly this is only rough, because not all cats have all the properties that are typical of cats; but each natural kind is constituted by a clustering of properties which approximates to the description given. Whether there are natural kinds in this sense is an empirical question (Mackie, 1976, p.87).

Thus we can say that properties A, B and C cluster if and only if the probability of finding any one of them in an object is enhanced given the fact that the object has one (or more) of the others. In order to provide a criterion of when a group of objects with a cluster of properties count as a (distinct) natural kind, we have to given the fact that the object has one (or more) of the others. In groups of objects exist in nature and are not arbitrarily created by cluster of properties counts as a (distinct) natural kind, we have to

The basic idea here is that intermediate sorts of objects should be relatively rare. If we take objects to be represented by points on a multidimensional character space, then a group of objects constitutes a natural kind (on this view) if and only if these points themselves cluster and intermediate points between neighbouring clusters are rare. On this view we can explain why a division of objects by size does not mark a natural kind – mapping such objects onto our multi-dimensional space we do have a boundary of rare intermediate forms. For a kind to constitute a natural kind, the objects must both share a cluster of properties, and there must be rarities or intermediate forms. As Brian Everitt puts it:

> A description of what constitutes a cluster which probably agrees closely with our intuitive understanding of the term is given by considering entities as points in a p-dimensional space, with each of the p-variables [properties] being represented by one of the axes of this space. The variable values for each entity now define a p-dimensional co-ordinate in this space. Clusters may now be described as continuous regions of this space containing a relatively high density of points, separated from other such regions by regions containing a relatively low density of points. Clusters described in this way are sometimes referred to as *natural clusters* (Everitt, 1980, p.60).

So this view can explain why large diamonds do not constitute a distinct natural kind from small diamonds. This is because even though there is more than one way of drawing the distinction between large and small diamonds (for example, by either size or mass), and so we could say that these sizes and masses clustered, the objects that are large diamonds do not form a distinct cluster of objects from small diamonds if mapped onto a multi-dimensional character space. Only if there are rare intermediate forms can we argue that we have distinct natural kinds.

However, this theory will not do either. This is because of the possibility of accidental kinds. Suppose that, quite by chance, all the objects in the world that have a certain bizarre shape, also have other properties in common – they have the same colour, the same mass, and so on. That is, suppose these objects (call them 'brutons') share a cluster of properties. Suppose too that when we map brutons onto a multi-dimensional character space, they form a distinct cluster of objects.

But we do not think that brutons form a natural kind because we know it is just an accident that they share this cluster of properties. One object may have been shaped by weather conditions out of granite stone, another might have been carved out of a piece of wood and painted, and so on. Although in each case there is an explanation how each object came to acquire those properties, the explanation in each case is different. Because there is no common explanation why brutons share the properties that they do, we take it to be an accident that they share such properties.

## (3) The explanatory nature criterion

On this theory, objects that share a cluster of properties only belong to the same natural kind if they share the same explanatory nature or real essence. This theory will explain why it is that the objects that accidentally share a cluster of characteristics (for example, brutons) do not constitute a natural kind.

It is not necessary for members of two different kinds to have any natural boundary (of rare intermediate forms) when these members are mapped onto a multi-dimensional character space. This is because if these members have a different explanatory nature, then even if they share the same cluster of observable properties, they belong to different natural kinds. Chromosomal doubling (polyploidy) can generate morphologically identical but distinct species of plant. They share the same cluster of morphological properties, but they nevertheless belong to distinct natural kinds in virtue of their having distinct genetic natures which keep them reproductively isolated (Mayr, 1963, p.20).

Conversely, the existence of distinct clusters of particulars in a multi-dimensional character space is not sufficient for the existence of two distinct natural kinds. In spite of the fact that male and female mallards have distinct clusters of properties, so much so that Linnaeus classified them into the two distinct species which he

37

named *Anas boschas* and Anas *platyrhnchos*, they belong to the same (species) natural kind (Mayr, 1963, p.22).

However, this account is not necessary for something to be a natural kind. There is the possibility of brute kinds – natural kinds that do not have explanatory natures at all (William Newton-Smith in conversation). We have found that the properties of animals are explained by a molecular nature, and that the properties of molecules are explained by an atomic nature, and that the properties of atoms are explained by a nuclear nature, and so on. This regress can end in a number of ways.

Firstly, in what I call the Chinese Box Universe, the regress might be infinite, and every kind might have an internal structure, composed of parts with their own internal structure in turn, and so on *ad infinitum*. Secondly, in what I call the Foundationless Universe, the regress might end with clusters of properties that simply lack any internal nature that explains why such properties cluster.

Let me illustrate this with the natural kind of electrons. Electrons have a cluster of properties – they share a negative charge, a particular mass, and a particular spin. In the Chinese Box Universe, electrons are, let us suppose, composed of poo-ons, which have a cluster of properties, and which in combination explain why electrons have the properties that they do. The cluster of properties of poo-ons in turn is explained by their internal structure, which consists of pee-ons. And so on. In the Foundationless universe, let us suppose that electrons are ultimate particles. They have a cluster of properties, but they do not have any internal structure that explains why they have the cluster of properties that they do. The regress of structures ends with the electron.

It is possible that we live in a Foundationless Universe, and that electrons are ultimate particles that have no internal structure. In fact, the current scientific view of electrons is that they have no structure at all. But electrons are paradigmatic examples of natural kinds even in our universe. And hence we cannot give an account of natural kinds in terms of the possession of explanatory natures.

There seem to be two possible sorts of natural kinds – Complex Kinds, comprised of objects that share an explanatory nature which explains their cluster of properties, and Ultimate Kinds, comprised of objects that share a cluster of properties but which do not share an explanatory nature because they all lack one. But if we admit that electrons constitute a natural kind simply in virtue of the fact that they share a distinct cluster of properties, we will have to regard accidental kinds such as brutons as natural kinds.

The account is not sufficient either if we adopt a certain view of explanation. On the standard account of explanation, we explain a fact by deducing a proposition describing it from propositions describing initial conditions and a law of nature (Hempel, 1965, p.247). On this view, laws of nature are true universal generalizations such as 'All electrons have a negative electrical charge.' However, there may be accidentally true universal generalizations that are not laws of nature. And if these are accepted as laws, we will have to admit bogus natural kinds.

Suppose it is an accidental fact that there are no lumps of gold or silver or copper in the universe greater than one million kilograms. These are accidental facts because if we were foolish enough to take the generalizations seriously, we could refute them by constructing such masses, and thereby prove they are not laws of nature.

Nevertheless, on this view of explanation, they are laws. So we have a clustering of the (negative) properties of not being gold, not being copper, and not being silver in objects greater than one million kilograms. And for such clusters, there is an explanatory nature which explains why the properties cluster – all such objects have a mass of greater than one million kilograms. Unless we can exclude such generalizations from being laws, we have to accept that masses greater than one million kilograms constitute natural kinds on this account.

## (4) The law-like connectedness criterion

On this theory, members belong to a natural kind if and only if they possess a cluster of properties, and these properties are connected to one another in the same way. That is, each member must have the same cluster of properties, and these properties must be associated in each member because of the same laws of nature.

Ultimate kinds like electrons are natural kinds because they have a cluster of properties (of charge, mass and spin) and because these properties are connected by the same ultimate laws of nature. An 'ultimate' law of nature is a regularity which cannot be explained by any more fundamental law. The connection between the negative charge of the electron and its spin is an ultimate law, for example, because it is a regularity of the universe which cannot be explained by any more basic law.

Of course, if the connection between the properties of an electron does not constitute an ultimate law of nature, but is explained by a more fundamental law, this will in no way change the status of electrons as natural kinds. With the discovery of a more basic explanation, electrons will still be a kind with a cluster of properties shown to be associated by the same (newly discovered) law of nature.

Complex kinds like gold are natural kinds because members have the same cluster of properties (of colour, density, etc.), and because the connection between such properties is explained by the same laws of nature (operating on the same internal nature). That is, the atomic nature of gold plus laws of physics together explain why any lump of gold has its unique cluster of properties.

On the other hand, accidental kinds like brutons are not natural kinds. Even though they have a cluster of properties, the connection between the cluster is accidental – the association is not explained by any laws of nature. Other kinds are not natural even though the cluster of properties possessed by members is not accidental – if members do not possess the same nature, they will not belong to the same natural kind.

For example, all pieces of jade share a cluster of common features, and although the properties in this cluster are not accidentally associated, what explains their possession differs from one piece of jade to the next. Hilary Putnam remarks:

> Although the Chinese do not recognize the difference, the term 'jade' applies to two minerals: jadeite and nephrite.
> Chemically, there is a marked difference. Jadeite is a combination of sodium and aluminium. Nephrite is made of calcium, magnesium and iron. These two quite different microstructures produce the same unique textural qualities (Putnam, 1976b, p.241)!

Because there is no common nature to jadeite and nephrite that explains their common jade-like properties, the same explanation why members have the cluster of properties does not hold of all pieces of jade. And hence jade is not a natural kind.

Of course, natural kinds do not have to have exactly the same natures to count as natural kinds. Acids have different natures in that they are different chemical compounds, but they all share the same nature of being proton-donors (or electron-pair acceptors) that explains the cluster of acidic properties.

Masses greater than 1 million kg also do not constitute a natural kind – they constitute another accidental kind. They might have a cluster of (negative) properties, and the 'explanation' for the clustering might be the same in each case, but the connection between the properties is not explained by any laws of nature. The generalizations that 'explain' why such properties cluster (for example, the generalization 'Everything with a mass greater than 1 million kg is not gold') are merely accidental generalizations and not laws of nature. And hence the connection between the (negative) properties is not explained by a law of nature.

Natural kinds are (by definition) groups that somehow exist independently of our classifications, and are the sort of thing that we can discover. We can see now why a definition employing the notion of laws of nature satisfies this requirement. Laws of nature are the sort of thing that exist independently of us and which we can discover. And hence natural kinds become the sort of thing that exist independently of us and which we can discover.

While this tells us *what* kinds are natural kinds, it does not tell us when natural kinds are *distinct*. To ensure that the requirement for the discoverability of natural kinds is preserved, we must require there to be natural boundaries between distinct natural kinds. Ultimate kinds have natural boundaries between one another if and only if the clusters of properties defining them are distinct. We have seen that clusters are distinct if and only if there is a relative rarity of intermediate forms. For example, positrons are a distinct natural kind from electrons because there is a rarity of intermediate forms – particles are not more or less positrons or more or less electrons.

Complex kinds have natural boundaries if and only if there are qualitative differences among their respective natures, or if the differences are only quantitative, they are not continuous. For example, different species belong to different natural kinds because their genetic natures are qualitatively distinct. And different elements belong to different natural kinds because although the differences between their atomic structures are quantitative – they all have a different number of positrons in their nuclei – the differences are not continuous. Any element is not more or less gold, or more or less silver – there are no intermediate forms.

On the other hand, different cloud genera do not form distinct natural kinds because there are no natural boundaries among their natures. Whether a cloud is a cumulus cloud rather than a stratus cloud depends on the degree of convectional currents in its nature (convectional currents explain why it is that cumulus clouds can produce hail – such currents re-cycle ice particles and give them a number of layers of ice). But there is no natural boundary between the natures of cumulus and stratus clouds – any intermediate can occur (there is even an intermediate genus known as stratocumulus clouds). Because there is no non-arbitrary point where a stratus cloud ends and a cumulus or a stratocumulus cloud begins, we cannot defend the idea that cloud genera are natural kinds and exist independently of our taxonomies.

A natural kind can then be defined thus:

> Objects belong to a distinct natural kind if and only if (1) they have the same cluster properties, (2) the possession of the cluster is explained in the same way (by the same laws of nature), and (3) natural boundaries exist between them and members of neighbouring kinds.

This account of natural kinds leaves us with the problem of distinguishing between laws of nature and accidental generalizations. However, solving this problem would take us beyond the scope of this book. What I hope I have shown is that the notion of natural kinds stands and falls with the notion of laws of nature. In addition, laws of nature will have to be more than simply true universal generalizations, otherwise we will have to admit bogus natural kinds like objects with masses greater than 1 million kg.

It is worth noting that ultimate kinds are clearly different from complex kinds. This can be seen from the fact that we have less of a grip on the idea that a single ultimate kind can take different forms. We can understand what it is for a complex kind to have a number of different forms. For these forms to be forms of a single kind they must share the same explanatory nature. Such a move is not available to us with ultimate kinds. How could we show that neutrinos, positrons, and muons were really electrons, if they all lack explanatory natures?

The identity conditions of the two sorts of kinds are different. Some form will count as the same complex kind as another form if and only if they share the same explanatory nature. But all ultimate kinds share the same explanatory nature, or lack of it. But this does not mean that all ultimate kinds are forms of the same natural kind. Rather, some form will count as the same ultimate kind if and only if it possesses the same cluster of properties.

Note that on this account of natural kinds, members do not have to be more similar to one another than to non-members in order to constitute a natural kind. In fact the account of natural kinds in terms of similarity raises a skeptical issue over the existence of natural kinds. As Evan Fales puts it:

> In its most general terms, skepticism about the existence of natural kinds poses the question of the very intelligibility of the claim that the members of one class of particulars are 'more similar' to each other than to any of the members of the second class, and vice versa. What can be meant in this context by 'more similar'? Clearly, no answer to this question will be forthcoming in terms of relative numbers of properties possessed by both members of any pair of particulars, or even by some measure of degrees of property-similarity. We sense that red is more similar to orange than to blue: but a general measure of property similarity eludes us, as does any technique for finitely enumerating the distinct objective monadic properties of particulars. If particulars have indefinitely many properties, then comparisons which utilize simple ratios of identical properties to non-identical ones cannot be made (Fales, 1982, p.69).

If we made the assumption that members have to be more similar to one another than to non-members, we would not be able to recognize the kinds that we do. For example, acids constitute a natural kind, but the members are not more similar to one another than to non-members. It may be that some acids share more properties with chemicals that are *not* acids. However, the important matter is whether all acids share a cluster of (acidic) properties which can be explained by some nature, rather than their overall similarity.

Because of this account of natural kinds, then, we can avoid such skeptical arguments about similarity. In addition, it becomes possible for one particular to be a member of a number of different natural kinds. One sample of stuff can be both a member of the chemical natural kind HCl, as well as being a member of the broader natural kind of acids. Similarly, an organism can be a member of a species natural kind, as well as a member of a genus natural kind. And hydrogen can be a member of an isotope natural kind as well as a member of an element natural kind.

A Taxonomic Skeptic might argue that what natural kinds we come to recognize is not something that is independent of us and the concepts with which we start describing and classifying objects. If the kinds we recognize are dependent on the concepts we possess, we cannot give any content to the idea that there are natural divisions among objects that our taxonomies, however they begin, can converge upon. He may argue that if we start with different concepts, we would arrive at different natural kinds. This, if it were true, would undermine the whole idea that there are natural kinds that exist independently of our attempts to recognize them.

Suppose we started out to describe the world with grue-concepts. Instead of describing things as green and blue, we would describe them as grue – something is grue if and only if it is green if the time is before AD 2000 and blue if the time is after AD 2000, and bleen – something is bleen if and only if it is blue if the time is before AD 2000 and green if the time is after AD 2000. Grue things change colour (from green to blue) at the time AD 2000, and bleen things change from blue to green. However, they do not change 'shmolor' – they remain grue and bleen over this period.

If we started with such descriptive concepts, we would recognize emerires and sapheralds as natural kinds, because in this conceptual scheme they (and not emeralds and sapphires) would share natures that explain their clusters of properties. Something is an emerire if and only if it has the nature of an emerald if the time is before AD 2000, and the nature of a sapphire if the time is after AD 2000. And conversely for sapheralds.

We might think that such kinds are really combinations of different kinds because we construct them out of different kinds, and that emerires at different times do not really share the same natures and properties. But someone with the grue-conceptual scheme can say the same of emeralds and sapphires as he defines them in terms of his concepts. According to him, something is an emerald if and only if it has the nature of an emerire if the time is before AD 2000, and the nature of a sapherald if the time is after AD 2000.

But if our grue-scientist convinces us that he does indeed have an alternative taxonomy to ours, we can only conclude that we cannot (prior to AD 2000) *discover* which taxonomy correctly identifies the natural kinds that exist in the world. The grue-scientist claims that there are emerires (and not emeralds), and therefore predicts that emerires will change colour at AD 2000 (though they will not change 'shmolor' – they will remain grue while they change colour from green to blue). Now if the stones in question do not change colour, then we will have reason to believe that the world contains the natural kinds of emeralds and not that of emerires. It need not be part of any theory about natural kinds that one will always be able to tell just which theory picks out the natural kinds we take to exist independently of us. In this case, prior to AD 2000, there is just no way to tell what natural kinds there are.

So we need not infer from this that what natural kinds we recognize depends on the concepts that we have. We only recognize different kinds because we are ignorant – when all the evidence is in, our taxonomies will converge. Should the stones change colour at AD 2000, perhaps we will accept that there are emerires rather than emeralds after all. The example we have given show that as we learn more about the world competing taxonomies converge on the one that picks out the existing natural kinds. And hence it does not show that what natural kinds we arrive at depends in any crucial way on the concepts that we have.

The skeptic may then argue that any theory is underdetermined by all actual and possible data. A theory is underdetermined by all actual data if and only if there is another conflicting theory that can also account for the same actual data. Suppose all the swans that we have so far observed have been white. We might formulate a theory that all swans are white. This theory is underdetermined by all actual data because there is another theory – all the swans in England are white, but there are some black swans in Australia – that also fits the actual data, but has conflicting predictions about the swans in Australia. The actual data underdetermines which theory is correct. But the theories are not underdetermined by all actual and possible data because there is some possible data – about swans in Australia – which will decide among them.

A theory is underdetermined by all actual *and* possible data if there is no data that could settle whether it or a competing theory were correct. For example, after the Michelson–Morley experiment failed to detect the ether, scientists eventually came to accept Einstein's theory that claimed that the ether did not exist. However, there was another theory (elaborated by Lorentz) which accounted for the same actual and possible data. This was the theory that there is an ether, but that objects contract as they move in the ether, and that clocks slow down as they move in the ether. These consequences of motion in the ether make the ether physically impossible to detect. And hence there is no way to decide which theory is right – the theories are underdetermined by all actual and possible data.

There are two responses to the position of underdetermination of theory by data (Newton-Smith, 1981, p.42). The Arrogance Response assumes that in such cases there simply is no fact of the matter at stake. In the example discussed, the world is not rich enough to contain either the fact that there is an ether, or the fact that there is no ether. The Ignorance Response, on the other hand, assumes that there is such a fact – it is just that we poor human beings do not have a rich enough cognitive and perceptual apparatus to gain access to such facts.

If all theories were underdetermined by all actual and possible data, and we assumed that there was a fact of the matter at stake, we would never be able to tell which theory was correct. If this applies to theories about what groups are natural kinds, we could never tell which theory successfully identified the independently existing natural kinds. If we wanted to defend TR, we would have to claim that there were indeed natural kinds, but that we could never find out what they were.

In such a case it would seem more plausible to adopt the Arrogance Response. However, the skeptic has not defended the main premise of the argument that all theory *is* underdetermined by all actual and possible data. It is not an easy task to produce genuine alternative theories (as opposed to a mere notational variant) to every theory that predicts exactly the same observations in all possible circumstances. And until this has been done, we need not take the skeptic seriously.

Thus we can make sense of the idea that there are natural kinds existing independently of our taxonomies, and which can be mirrored by them. Whether there are natural kinds is an empirical matter, and we have good reason to believe that there are many natural kinds. Isotopes, elements, chemicals, biological species, etc. all seem to qualify. All members have clusters of properties connected to one another by the same laws of nature. The atomic essence of each element explains in the same way why members have the same cluster of properties. The molecular essence of each chemical explains in the same way why members have the same cluster of properties. The genetic essence of each biological species explains in the same way why members have the same cluster of traits. And so on.

Of course, not all kinds we recognize are natural kinds. Trees probably do not constitute a natural kind. Most trees have ovaries and belong to the natural kind of angiosperms, while some like pine trees do not – trees do not share a common explanatory nature in virtue of which they constitute a higher order natural kind. Whether or not a plant is a tree depends not on its nature but on its general form (Dupré, 1981, p.89).

But as long as there are some natural kinds, some sense can be made of the Taxonomic Realists' claim that taxonomies can be correct (if they mirror such natural kinds) or incorrect (if they do not). We must now investigate the second tenet of TR – that our terms can purport to pick out such natural kinds.

# CHAPTER 3
# TAXONOMIC REALISM 2: SEMANTICS

## Introduction

I have argued that we can make sense of the idea of natural kinds existing independently of our attemps to classify objects. And that natural kinds exist – gold, tigers, water, electrons, and so on. But in order for us to be able to make the further claim that our taxonomies can be correct or incorrect, we must argue that our terms purport to pick out natural kinds. If we accepted that there were natural kinds, but never intended our taxonomies to reflect such natural divisions, then there would be no sense in which such taxonomies could be in error. It is only if they purport to pick out such kinds that they can be in error when they fail to correspond to them. If our terms only purport to express nominal essences, and not pick out natural kinds, then our taxonomies cannot be convicted of being incorrect. They can be more or less useful, but this is another matter.

If for example I classify plants into shrubs, trees, creepers, herbs, and so on and it is pointed out to me that such a taxonomy does not categorize things into natural kinds, I need not thereby concede that my taxonomy is mistaken. It may not be very useful, but that is another thing. If the terms (like 'tree') never purported to pick out natural kinds, then the taxonomy is not mistaken for not doing so. In order for TR to be correct, classificatory terms must purport to pick out natural kinds. In this chapter I will examine the semantics of our classificatory terms and see whether they do indeed purport to pick out natural kinds.

## Semantic theories

In order for a term to purport to pick out a natural kind, it must

48

have what I will call a Natural Kind Semantics (NKS for short). One possible way for terms to have an NKS is for them to refer to real essences – objects grouped on the basis of sharing a real essence will constitute a natural kind. Alternatively, if terms have what I will call a Descriptive Semantics (DS for short), they may not group objects into natural kinds. One possible way for terms to have a DS is for them to express nominal essences, but if objects are grouped on such a basis, we know that many such collections will not constitute natural kinds.

For example, if 'gold' purports to pick out the real essence of gold, it will classify lumps into a natural kind. Anything that has the explanatory nature of gold will be gold, and such a class will constitute a natural kind. On the other hand, if 'gold' means 'something that is yellow, malleable, shiny, etc.', then objects will not necessarily be grouped into natural kinds. Substances with different natures, like fool's gold, but with the same observable properties enumerated in the descriptive definition, will fall into the same (non-natural) kind.

There are basically two sorts of relations that can exist between objects and the terms that purport to pick them out. The first relation is Semantical, the second Causal. The relation is semantical when the term picks out the object if and only if the object *satisfies* some description that the term expresses. Terms with a DS have this sort of relation with objects they classify. The relation is causal when the term picks out the object if and only if there is some appropriate causal relation between the object and the term. Terms with an NKS have this sort of relation with the objects they classify.

There are two DS theories that I will examine. One I will call the Nominal Essence Theory, and the other the Family Resemblance Theory. There are two NKS theories that I will be looking at. One I will call the Causal Theory, and the other the Combined Theory. I will first give an account of these theories, and then go on to see what meaning our actual terms have.

Until the 1950s, there was only one general theory about the meaning of our terms. This is what I have called the Nominal Essence Theory, and it was put forward by Goetlieb Frege and Bertrand Russell. The basic idea is that the meaning of a term consists in the expression of those properties that make up the nominal essence of that kind. The nominal essence consists in those properties by which members of that kind are standardly recognized. On this theory, then 'gold' means 'substance that is yellow, malleable, shiny, etc.'. The extension of a kind term is determined by the description that members of that kind have to satisfy.

Ludwig Wittgenstein then added another theory – the Family Resemblance Theory. On the Nominal Essence Theory, members of a kind have to satisfy all the predicates which are taken to be jointly necessary and sufficient for membership. But Wittgenstein argued that many of our classificatory terms do not have a set of predicates the satisfaction of which is jointly necessary and sufficient for membership. Instead, members need only satisfy a proportion of the predicates – they bear family resemblances to one another.

In families, all members do not have the family nose, the family chin, the family ears, and so on. But all have a significant proportion of them so that they are recognizably of the same family. Similarly, some terms like 'game' do not express nominal essences – all games do not have winners and losers, more than one player, the requirement of some skill on the part of the players, and so on. But all games satisfy a proportion of such a set of predicates that makes them games – they are connected by family resemblances. The term 'game' does not express a nominal essence, but only family resemblances.

Note that if our terms had a DS, TR would be false. As I have argued, if classificatory terms express nominal essences, then we cannot convict the taxonomy of error – it is not trying to pick out natural kinds, and so is not mistaken if it happens not to do so. And because what lines we wish to draw depend on us, there is a sense in which we invent the kinds that are found in our taxonomies rather than discover them. If we want to include whales with salmon, trout, etc., all we have to do is to adopt a definition of 'fish' as 'aquatic vertebrate'. If we do not, all we do is adopt a different definition of 'fish': it is up to us. The same argument applies to terms that express family resemblances.

In the 1970s, two philosophers independently developed an alternative semantic theory for some of our terms. Hilary Putnam and Saul Kripke put forward what I have called the Causal Theory. The idea was simple but radical – terms in our taxonomies do not have any descriptive meaning at all! Instead, they have a reference – they refer to the real essences of objects. The extension of a term is not determined by the nominal essence of that kind, that is, the cluster of properties by which members of that kind are standardly recognized. Rather, the extension is determined by the possession of the same explanatory nature as possessed by some member that stands in the right sort of causal relation to our use of that term. The extension is thus determined by whatever objects have the same nature as that object referred to by our term.

The idea is that we come across a sample object, like a piece of gold. We do not define 'gold' by listing those predicates like 'yellow' that pieces of gold have to satisfy. For to do this might mean that we do not pick out a natural kind – it may be that fool's gold also satisfies these predicates. Instead, we define 'gold' in terms of whatever other objects share the same nature as *this* sample – that is, share the same nature as the stuff causally connected to the use of our term 'gold'. The sample is causally connected in that it is causally responsible for our awareness of that object and for our invocation of a name to call that sort of object. Even if we do not (yet) know what this nature consists in, we can commit ourselves to only calling those things gold that share the same nature as *this*. This means that we can pick out a natural kind even though we do not know what nature all such members of that kind share (in the case of gold, they all have 79 protons in their nucleus).

There is another theory for terms with the NKS – I will call it the Combined Theory. Here objects belong to the same kind if they satisfy a minimal description of what sort of object they are, and if they stand in the right sort of causal relation to our use of the term. Thus, in order to know the meaning of a term, like 'gold', one has to grasp that gold is a substance – this is the minimal descriptive meaning of the term. However, unlike the DS theories, this description is not sufficient to fix the extension of the kind. This is achieved by the causal component of the Combined Theory. *Which* substance we are picking out is determined by the possession of the same explanatory nature as possessed by those objects that stand in the right sort of causal relation to our use of the term.

## What language do we speak?

These different theories give an account of possible languages that can be spoken. We need to discover which of these possible languages is the one that we speak. It is not enough to know what meanings our classificatory terms *could* have – we must find out what meanings they *actually* have.

51

There are three arguments standardly given which purport to show that classifactory terms in our lanaguage do not have a DS. After Nathan Salmon, these will be known as the Metaphysical, the Epistemological, and the Semantical arguments (Salmon, 1982, pp.22–31). However, since the first two arguments depend crucially on what we mean by our terms, we could say that all the arguments are in a sense Semantical.

The Metaphysical argument is this: If 'tiger' means 'animal that is striped, cat-like, etc.', then it is not possible for something to be a tiger and lack any or all of these properties – it is a self-contradiction to say a striped animal is not striped. But it *does* seem possible for tigers to lack some of these properties. Tigers might acquire a dreadful viral disease *in utero* that suppresses the expression of certain tiger-genes, so that they develop into different-looking creatures, lacking many of their definitional properties. But they would still be tigers, albeit diseased ones.

According to the Epistemological argument, it is possible that we could discover that the animals we call 'tigers' do not have the properties we take to constitute their nominal essence. That is, it is possible that we discover that their striped skin is due to a vitamin-deficiency disease, which upon correction disappears. But this would not amount to the discovery that tigers did not exist, but only that tigers were not striped. But if 'tiger' meant 'striped animal', this discovery would not be possible. Therefore, 'tiger' does not have a DS.

The Semantical argument proceeds thus: It could turn out that the creatures we have been calling tigers are cleverly disguised robots from Mars, and that there is (unbeknown to us) on some remote planet in the galaxy some organisms satisfying the description believed true of tigers. If our terms had a DS, we would have to say we were talking about the organisms on the remote planet, and not about the robots. But this seems implausible – it seems that we are talking about the robots (and believing many false things of them), rather than talking about a class of objects that is totally unrelated to us and that by chance satisfies the definition of 'tiger'.

At this stage it is worth noting that these arguments are only aimed at showing that the meaning of our classificatory terms cannot be descriptive. They do not show what meaning they actually possess. In addition, the arguments are flawed in an important way. They depend for their success on what we would say, that is, on our linguistic intuitions. But in order to see what semantic theory applies to our classificatory terms, we ought ideally to test the whole community's intuitions. Only in this way could we discover what theory is correct about our *common* language. It may be that the Causal Theory is the best account of Putnamese, but the important issue is what language the rest of us speak.

Let us return to the arguments. It will now be apparent that they are not conclusive, for it is open to us to say that other creatures with a different nature but the same tiger-like appearance *would* be tigers, or that if tigers lost their present observable properties, they would *not* be tigers. So these arguments do not show that our terms do not have a DS.

Hilary Putnam puts forward two arguments that purport to show that our terms have a meaning as outlined by the Causal Theory. However, these are flawed for a similar reason. The first runs like this: We may discover on Mars a substance with all the phenomenal properties of water but having the different theoretical nature of XYZ (instead of $H_2O$). Hilary Putnam uses this example to argue that since we would not call such a stuff 'water', the extension of the term is determined by what possesses the same theoretical nature as the stuff (on earth) that stands in the right sort of causal relation to our use of the term, and not by the superficial observable properties of water (Putnam, 1976b, pp.223-5).

However, Eddy Zemach points out that this simply begs the question that XYZ is not (a form of) water. When we discover that the nature of Martian liquid is XYZ, instead of saying that we had discovered that it was not water, we might instead say that we had discovered that water was not a natural kind (Zemach, 1976, p.120). Just as we have discovered that jade is not a natural kind because pieces of jade can have different theoretical natures and not share any common theoretical nature, so we can discover that water is not a natural kind. So it seems that Hilary Putnam's example is not conclusive. His intuitions might lead him to say that XYZ is not water, but the rest of us might have intuitions which would lead us to classify XYZ as (a form of) water.

The other argument Hilary Putnam uses to support the Causal Theory is about cats. He supposes that some objects we call 'cats' turn out to be robot cats from Mars. Because most of us would feel that the Martian robots were not cats, this seems to show that 'cat' does not have a DS, but instead a meaning given by the Causal Theory (Putnam, 1976a, pp.238-9). However, it might be argued that if 'cat' expresses the nominal essence 'animal that is furry, cat-like, etc.', this would explain why the Martian robots are not cats, because they are not animals!

The moral of the story is that we should set aside personal linguistic intuitions to support the different theories, and turn instead to the actual use of terms to see what meaning they have. When we do that, we find evidence that our scientific terms have an NKS as outlined by the Combined Theory. The evidence can be divided into five sorts of cases – exclusion or inclusion of borderline cases, existential assertions, existential denials, identity judgments, and ambiguous reference.

The exclusion of fool's gold from being an instance of gold provides support for some NKS theory over some DS theory. Even though fool's gold might satisfy the nominal essence or descriptive meaning of 'gold', it is not gold because it does not have the same theoretical nature of the stuff that stands in the right sort of causal relation to our use of the term 'gold'. It is because the nature of fool's gold does not consist in having an atomic structure of 79 protons that it is not gold.

Similarly, the inclusion of graphite with diamond as instances of the element carbon supports the view that our terms have an NKS rather than a DS. In spite of the fact that the nominal essence of diamond and graphite are different, they are instances of the same element carbon because the nature that stands in the right sort of causal relation to the use of each term is the same.

Evidence from existential assertions also supports the view that our terms have an NKS. After it was discovered that the electron did not have the sort of properties Niels Bohr had supposed it to have (like a definite position and momentum at any one time), it was not concluded that the electron did not exist (because nothing satisfied the definitional description of the term 'electron'). Rather, it was concluded that the electron existed, but failed to have the properties it was believed to have. Anything was an electron if it stood in the right sort of causal relation to Bohr's use of the term in relation to such things as cathode rays. These sorts of cases are good support for the theory that our terms have an NKS.

Priestley and other eighteenth-century chemists held that when metals such as mercury and tin were burned in air (that is, oxidized – a process they called 'calcination'), phlogiston was given off. The metal had collapsed into a powder (that is, an oxide, but which they called 'calx') upon losing phlogiston. The metal could be restored from the calx by restoring phlogiston to it, which could be achieved when the calx was reacted with coke (in other words, reduced). The term 'phlogiston' stands in the right sort of casual relation to the lack of oxygen. But this does not mean that they were talking all along about the absence of oxygen, and the phlogiston exists after all! In spite of the fact that the lack of oxygen stands in the right sort of causal relation to their use of the term 'phlogiston', 'phlogiston' was not referring to this *absence*, but was rather intended to refer to some *substance*. This is evident from the fact that when it was discovered that the addition of phlogiston to the substance resulted in that substance having a smaller mass, it was thought that phlogiston must have a negative mass.

On the Causal Theory, it is difficult to obtain a *failure* of reference, and in this case commits us to saying that phlogiston exists after all. However, it is clear that we all think that phlogiston does not exist, and this is because it is part of the descriptive meaning of the term 'phlogiston' that it is a substance (and not just the absence of something else). It is because there is nothing *of that description* that stands in the right sort of causal relation to their use of the term 'phlogiston', that we say that phlogiston does not exist. If we already have evidence for some NKS theory, this sort of example supports the Combined Theory over the Causal Theory.

The example does not support the theory that our terms have a DS. When Niels Bohr talked about electrons, he took them to have properties (like a definite position and momentum at any time) which they do not have. But we still take him to have been talking about the electron because there was something that both satisfied the description of being a particle and that stood in the right sort of causal relation to his use of the term. Only some features of the description are necessarily true of an electron, and not all.

Similarly, astronomers in the nineteenth century pointed their telescopes towards Mercury and thought they had discoverd a new planet which they called 'Vulcan'. However, it turned out that what was in the right sort of causal relation to their use of this term was not a planet, but a sunspot. On the Causal Theory, we would be forced to say that we did not discover that Vulcan did not exist, but rather that Vulcan had turned out to be a sunspot! It seems clear that what we *did* say was that Vulcan did not exist, and so it seems clear that we do not speak Causalese. On the other hand, the Combined Theory can explain why we say that Vulcan does not exist – the object that stands in the right sort of casual relation does not have the property (of being a planet or celestial body) which is the minimal descriptive component of the meaning of 'Vulcan'.

In addition, identity statements provide further evidence that our terms have a meaning as outlined by the Combined Theory and not the Causal Theory. The great entomologist, Uvarov, discovered that *Schistocerca gregaria* and *Schistocerca solitaria*, hitherto considered distinct species, were in fact simply seasonal forms of the same species. Here it was said that he had discovered that they were the same natural kind. But if we spoke Causalese, we would not say this. Suppose these seasonal variants have different natures (they must differ in some fundamental way which explains their superficial differences). Then the terms would *not* be picking out the same natural kind, and it would be *wrong* to say that they had been found to be identical. It is only if we assume that we are taking about a *species* (and not just seasonal variants) that we can claim (quite naturally) to have discovered that what we thought were members of a different kind were all along members of the same one. This supports the Combined Theory that takes such terms to carry the descriptive meaning that they are species.

There is another piece of evidence that we do not speak Causalese – it is too ambiguous. If we determine the extension of a term by those objects that possess *the* same explanatory nature as the object that stands in the right sort of causal relation to our use of the term, we will not have unambiguously picked out a single natural kind. Such an account of the meaning of the term provides us with no means of telling *which* natural kind we are talking about, because it provides us with no means of specifying *which* explanatory nature fixes the extension. If we define 'hydrogen' as that stuff with the same nature as *this*, it is not clear that we are referring to the nature of having so many protons in the nucleus, and hence talking about the element, or referring to the nature of having so many nucleons in the nucleus, and hence talking about the isotope. Similarly, if we encountered one species of elm tree, and used the name 'elm' to talk about the trees, it would not be clear whether we were talking about the species of elm or the genus. The only way of disambiguating the reference is if our terms have a minimal descriptive meaning that specifies whether we are talking about the species or genus. That is, our terms have to have a meaning as outlined by the Combined Theory.

It is worth noting that our ordinary proper names also seem to have a meaning as outlined by the Combined Theory. If I overhear a conversation about 'Lester Piggott', and learn that he has won nine Derbies, I do not grasp the meaning of the name unless I know that Lester Piggot is not a horse, but a man. If I think that he is a horse, I will not have grasped the meaning of the name. The descriptive content (namely, 'being a man') is part of the meaning of the name, but it is not sufficient to determine its reference. This is fixed by whatever man stands in the right sort of causal relation to the use of that name.

These examples from our actual use of classificatory terms seem to support the theory that the meaning of our terms is best explained by the Combined Theory. That is, they have an NKS. It is difficult (and I think impossible) to show that all our classificatory terms have such a semantics. I will show below that terms referring to ultimate kinds have a different semantics. In addition, not all terms classifying complex kinds have such a semantics. For example, terms like 'tree' do not purport to pick out natural kinds. As it has turned out, trees do not constitute a natural kind – it is because of the organism's *form* that it is classified as a tree. On discovering that trees do not constitute a natural kind, we do not conclude that there are no trees.

This example raises the first of two powerful philosophic arguments against the view that any of our terms have an NKS. Let us suppose that the term 'water' *does* have an NKS as outlined by the Causal Theory. Something is water, on this theory, if and only if it possesses *the* same nature as possessed by samples that stand in the right sort of causal relation to our use of the term. If 'water' has this meaning, and if we discover that water does not have a single common explanatory nature, we will have to conclude that there is no such thing as water. It is at least a possibility that this stuff does not have a common nature, but it is unlikely that we will ever conclude that there is no such thing as water. Rather, and more naturally, we will say that we have discovered that contrary to common belief, it has turned out that water is not a natural kind, but consists of a number of distinct natural kinds. Therefore, the term 'water' (and other such terms) has a descriptive meaning and not one given by the Causal Theory! As Eddy Zemach argues:

Is it so unreasonable to expect, then, that with further developments in science we may discover that on a more fundamental level some $H_2O$ molecules are essentially different from other $H_2O$ molecules? It may even be the case that, in the new classification, one kind of $H_2O$ molecule will turn out to be essentially closer to the XYZ molecule than to some other kind of $H_2$ molecule. What, then, will the reference of 'water' be? If Putnam's recommendations on the reference of substance-terms are adopted, we may have to reach the conclusion that there are no substance-terms in English at all (Zemach, 1976, p.121).

This does not mean that such kinds as water and chlorine are not natural kinds. Hugh Mellor argues:

> If Zemach's ... heavy water are too rare and exotic to convince, try the two common isotopes of chlorine. ... It is ... undeniable that the extension of 'chlorine' included both isotopes before their discovery, and so presumably includes both isotopes now. What Putnam must say is that chlorine and water have been found not to be natural kinds after all, but rather mixtures of natural kinds. But in that case, as Zemach ... observes, it will very likely turn out that we have no natural kind terms (Mellor, 1977, p.303).

But this does not follow at all. The existence of a number of isotopes of chlorine does not show that chlorine is not a natural kind. True, chlorine is a higher-order (elemental) natural kind that contains two lower-order (isotopic) natural kinds, but this does not show that the higher-order kind is not a natural kind. As long as the different isotopes share some explanatory nature that explains their possession of similar chemical properties, chlorine is a natural kind. And similarly with water. It is only when there is *no* common explanatory nature (as with jade) that we deny that we are dealing with a natural kind. We cannot infer from the fact that members of a natural kind do not have exactly the same nature that they do not constitute a natural kind. Different acids do not have the same nature – some are HCl, others $H_2SO_4$ – these do not have the same chemical structure, but it is because they share *some* nature that explains their acidic properties that acids count as a natural kind. Mark Platts remarks:

> But it simply does not follow that, for such physicists, chlorine has been found not to be a natural kind after all, but rather a mixture of natural kinds. The possibility remains open that

chlorine has been found to be a higher level natural kind relative to its isotopes. All that is needed for that to be defensible is that the isotopes of a given element share some property – plausibly, that recorded by the atomic number of the element – which is discovered both to serve to distinguish that kind from yet higher level kinds and also to be of importance for explanation of relevant kinds of physical properties (Platts, 1983, p.141).

So by admitting that members of the same kind have different natures (in some respect other than used to explain the shared properties) we are not admitting that there are no natural kinds. Of course, as I have argued, it is *possible* that we discover that there is no such natural kind as water, or even that none of our terms that purport to pick out natural kinds succeed in doing so. But because of the uniformity of nature, it is overwhelmingly *improbable* that most clusters of properties do not have a common explanatory nature. And so it is overwhelmingly improbable that no term with an NKS will successfully refer. Nevertheless, the argument is powerful support for some DS theory, because for many kinds we do not want to admit even the possibility that they might not exist, and if this is so, they cannot have an NKS.

But I do think that most of the classificatory terms that are used by scientists have such a semantics. This means that were we to discover that water is not a natural kind, we would have to conclude that there is no such thing as water. However, I think that what happens when such discoveries are made is that the terms *change* their meaning. When it is discovered that the objects picked out do not constitute a natural kind, one of two things can happen. We can conclude that there are no such things as Xs, and drop the term 'X', or we can retain the term 'X' but with a changed meaning, so that we continue to say that there are Xs.

What influences which alternative is adopted depends on how well entrenched the term is in the language. A term like 'water' is fairly well entrenched in our language, and so we would rather change its meaning than conclude that there is no such thing as water in the world. On the other hand, terms like 'phlogiston' or 'caloric' were not well entrenched in our language, and therefore we conclude that there are no such things when we discover that there is no natural kind in question. What such a theory has to do is to provide some means of showing that a term has *changed* its sense.

For why should we argue that the term 'water' has changed its sense to a purely descriptive meaning rather than its having had this meaning all along?

I think we can have evidence that some terms once had an NKS purporting to pick out a natural kind, but now have a DS. 'Fish' is one such term. To explain why people saw themselves as having discovered that whales were not fish when they discovered that whales had a mammalian nature, we have to assume that 'fish' had an NKS. However, in spite of the fact that it is now recognized that lungfish are closer to cows in origin (and hence share a genetic nature with cows rather than salmon), lungfish are still classified as fish. ('Fish is fish.') This seems to show that the term now has a DS – something is a fish if it has the form of a fish whatever its nature. That is, we have evidence that the term has changed its sense.

If we can make sense of the idea that terms with an NKS could change their sense, then we can indeed defend the idea that many of our terms classifying complex kinds have such a semantics. But there is a second argument against the claim that any of our terms have an NKS. This argument starts with the point that terms referring to ultimate kinds cannot have an NKS. This is because we have noted that they do not have any explanatory nature at all! If the extension of such a term is determined by whatever objects have the same nature as some sample object, our terms will either have no extension at all, or too wide an extension.

A term may have no extension at all because any sample ultimate kind will lack a nature, and so no objects can have the same nature as the sample. It may have too wide an extension if we consider that no nature is a sort of nature. If so, then every ultimate object (or any kind) – since they all lack natures – will fall under any term purporting to pick out an ultimate kind. So every ultimate kind will be identical! But this is absurd. This means that such terms have a different meaning, and a descriptive meaning seems the only possible one here.

This means that counter-factuals about ultimate particles will have a different logic. We can say, for example, that water could have different properties, because we can imagine a world where stuff composed of $H_2O$ has different surface properties. Similarly, we can claim that tigers might not have had stripes, because we can imagine a world where organisms with the genetic nature of tigers have a disease inhibiting the expression of the genes coding for stripes. But we cannot imagine a world where electrons have different properties (assuming that they do constitute an ultimate kind) because we cannot imagine a world where particles with the nature of electrons have different properties simply because electrons have no nature! This offers a serious objection for those who wish to argue that *all* our scientific terms have an NKS. Nevertheless, we can still argue that one such theory applies to complex kinds.

The argument is that we are never in a position to know whether a kind is an ultimate kind or a complex kind. If this is so, then none of our terms can have an NKS. If we take our terms to have an NKS, and if it is possible to discover that any complex kind is in fact an ultimate kind (because it lacks a nature), we have to accept the possibility that the supposed complex kind we are talking about either does not exist, or is identical to other ultimate kinds. But we are not prepared to tolerate the possibility that tigers do not exist, or that they are identical to electrons! Therefore, 'tiger' does not have an NKS.

In spite of this argument, we have seen that many of our terms behave just as if they have an NKS (of the Combined Theory sort). We could defend the view that these terms indeed have an NKS because in such cases we *do* know that the kinds have natures (and are not ultimate kinds). And if we do know that such kinds are not ultimate kinds, we have already excluded the possibility that tigers have the same nature – namely, none – as electrons, or that they do not exist.

In addition, we could always argue (as we did above) that our terms could start off with an NKS, and in the (unlikely) eventuality of the kind being an ultimate one, the meaning of the term could change to preserve the truth of sentences containing that term. Thus this argument too is not compelling.

If the arguments in this chapter have been convincing, I have shown that many of our terms have an NKS. That is, they purport to pick out natural kinds, and their extension is fixed by whatever both satisfies a minimal description as well as by whatever has the same real essence or explanatory nature as those objects that stand in the right causal relation to the use of the term. Because we often speak Combinese, that is, some language with an NKS, we have shown that TR may be true of any domain.

TR will not be true of all domains. We have pointed out that some taxonomies in everyday language – like the division of plants into trees, shrubs, herbs, and so on – do not purport to pick out natural kinds. In addition, there may be some specific scientific taxonomies that do not purport to pick out natural kinds. I suspect that most higher-order taxa in biology are not natural kinds, and that the terms in question do not purport to pick out the real essences of such kinds. It is most unlikely that all plants share a nature in virtue of which they are all plants. But I have not the space to argue for this conclusion here. Most importantly for our purposes, we have shown that TR may apply to any domain (we cannot exclude it out of hand), and that whether it does is something that we have to discover in each case.

# CHAPTER 4
# THE NATURE OF DISEASE

## Introduction

If you ask yourself what it is about a condition that makes it a disease, you might say: 'Something is a disease if it is a process of a certain sort, like an infection.' That is, we often think that something is a disease if it has a particular sort of nature. This response I will label the 'Essentialist Fallacy', so called because it assumes that being a disease consists in having a particular sort of nature. It is often made by laymen, and has been made in the history of the classification of diseases.

Towards the end of the nineteenth century, the Germ Theory of disease reached its height of popularity. The striking breakthroughs of Pasteur and Koch had persuaded many that all diseases were infections, and due to different germs. For example, the nutritional disease beriberi was also thought to be an infectious disease, and the search was on for the special bacterium. With this theory, many came to think that if a condition was an infection, then *ipso facto* it was a disease.

The same Germ Theory held sway in plant pathology too. Bacteria had been associated with plant disease since 1858, when Lachman observed bacteria in root nodules. In 1866, Woronin observed bacteria in the nodules of lupine. He concluded that this was a disease *because* it was due to a bacterial infection (Lechevalier and Solotorovsky, 1974, p.166). He made the Essentialist Fallacy – a condition was a disease in virtue of its nature.

The Essentialist Fallacy will be examined in this chapter – we will see whether all diseases share a particular sort of underlying nature. We will look at the medical category of disease and see whether there is any distinction between diseases on the one hand, and other pathological or negative medical conditions on the other. In addition, I will examine what sort of distinction it is.

It may be that diseases fall into a natural kind, and share a different real essence from other pathological conditions. This is what would have to be the case if TR were to apply to the domain of bodily conditions. On the other hand, it may be that diseases do not form a natural kind, and that they only share a nominal essence. Another alternative is that diseases do not share a nominal essence either, but instead share family resemblances with one another that are not shared by other pathological conditions. Finally, it may be that the category or disease is based upon a mistaken belief, and that there is no distinction at all between diseases and other negative medical conditions – only a *falsely believed* difference. (The distinction between pathological conditions and normality will occupy our attention in Chapter 5 – here I will be concerned only with the distinction *within* the broader class of pathological or negative medical conditions between those that are diseases and those that are not).

To illustrate these possibilities, let us look at the concept of 'fish'. Fish might fall into a single natural kind in virtue of sharing a 'fishy' nature not shared by other non-fishy animals. Or like jade, fish might not share the same explanatory nature – rather, they all share some nominal essence – perhaps they are all aquatic animals. Or fish might not even share a nominal essence, but rather are related by family resemblances. Finally, it might be that the distinction between fish and other animals is based on some mistaken belief. Perhaps we believe that there is some special as yet undiscovered property of 'fishiness' which we believe fish have and non-fish lack, so that when we discover there is no such property, we should abandon the distinction.

As I have suggested, it is possible that diseases form a natural kind. If this is so, we would have an easy solution to the many problems that we encountered earlier. We would be able to decide whether insurance companies should fund the treatment of stuttering, or whether the NHS should pay for the treatment of smoking, or whether we should sedate hyperactive children. All we would have to do is to see whether these conditions share the same nature (and thereby fall into the same natural kind) as conditions like TB, multiple sclerosis, breast cancer, and so on.

On the other hand, if diseases only share a nominal essence, whether homosexuality is a disease will depend on how one defines 'disease'. If 'disease' means 'deviant condition', then homosexuality will be a disease. It it means 'harmful deviant condition', it may well not be a disease. This solution to the problem of how to classify bodily conditions leaves unsolved the issue of what definition of disease to adopt. And so it would be useful if TR did apply to bodily conditions.

## Pathological conditions

There is a great variety of pathological or negative medical conditions – tuberculosis, schizophrenia, motion sickness, cerebral palsy, club foot, stroke, multiple sclerosis, myopia, albinism, lead poisoning, skull fracture, syphilis, sunburn, cleft palate, carbon-monoxide poisoning, drowning, diabetes mellitus, athlete's foot, lung cancer, Down's syndrome, fever, anaemia, migraine, cirrhosis, motor-neurone disease, mitral stenosis, frostbite, starvation, and so on. These conditions seem to fall into a number of mutually exclusive negative medical categories – not all of them are classified as diseases.

Some are diseases – tuberculosis, syphilis, schizophrenia, motor-neurone disease, multiple sclerosis, and lung cancer. Others are injuries – lacerations, gunshot wounds, burns, skull fracture. Someone with gunshot wounds does not have a disease (of lead poisoning!) – even though we may sometimes speak of them (in BBC English) as being 'critically ill'.

Then there are conditions that are classified as defects, disabilities, and/or deformities. We think of someone who is short-sighted as having a defect rather than having a disease. Similarly, we think of children with club foot, or cleft palate, as not being diseased, but rather as having some deformity. Finally, blind people are not thought of as diseased (although we accept that they might have had some disease which resulted in blindness), but rather as having some disability.

In medical discourse we make a distinction between those conditions that are merely signs, or symptoms, or even syndromes, rather than diseases. Thus fever is a sign of a disease, and not a disease itself. And weakness is a symptom of a disease, and not a disease. Similarly, the clinician never ceases to emphasize that conditions like anaemia are not diseases, but are rather signs of some underlying disease – 'Anaemia is not a diagnosis.' Even a condition like diabetes mellitus is said not to be a disease, but only a syndrome (a syndrome is a constellation or cluster of signs and symptoms):

Diabetes Mellitus is now accepted to be a syndrome rather than a single disease. The broad division into type I and II – that is, insulin-dependent and insulin-independent diabetes, irrespective of age of onset – is now widely recognized (Baltozzo *et al.*, 1978, p.1253).

What is classified as a sign, symptom, syndrome or disease varies with our increasing knowledge. Fever at one time was considered to be a disease entity, and so was diabetes mellitus. Now we tend to regard fever as just the manifestation of any number of different diseases – malaria, Hodgkin's disease, and so on. Similarly, we think of the syndrome of diabetes mellitus as the manifestation of any of a number of different diseases – insulin-dependent diabetes, insulin-independent diabetes, chronic pancreatitis, and so on. Thus what at one time may have been classified as a disease entity may later (with increasing knowledge) come to be classified differently. (Note that ordinary language classification might lag behind scientific language classification. What in ordinary discourse might be classified as a disease entity may no longer be so classified in medical discourse. For laymen, anaemia may well qualify as a disease entity, whereas this is not true in medical discourse.)

Then there are those conditions that are pathological states or lesions, for example, mitral stenosis and cirrhosis of the liver. These conditions are not disease entities either – rather they are viewed as pathological bodily states. They are, in essence, abnormal anatomical states that are observed by the pathologist and not the clinician.

There is a class of conditions not exclusive of disease which we might call poisonings. Some poisonings due to chemicals are classified as diseases by medical discourse, for example chronic lead poisoning. Others, like carbon-monoxide poisoning or barbiturate overdose, are not classified as diseases by either lay or medical discourse alike.

Finally, there is a rag-bag of conditions that do not fall into a neat medical category, but nevertheless fall under medical care. Conditions such as starvation, heat stroke, burns, motion sickness, and so on, are not regarded as diseases but are still negative medical conditions. Someone starving to death is not taken to have a disease, but is still not considered healthy.

Note that there are many conditions that are not classified as pathological conditions, but are considered part of normality.

Conditions like balding, the menopause, ageing, are normal and not pathological. The distinction between normality and conditions that one might broadly call abnormal or pathological will be the subject of Chapter 5 – I am concerned here only with the distinction *within* the class of pathological conditions between those that are diseases and those that are not.

These classes of negative medical conditions are recognized by medical and lay discourse alike. In fact, the classes recognized by the layman and the physician are largely identical, with medical classification of conditions as diseases being more liberal than the lay classification. In a study of such classificatory habits, conditions that were the result of some infectious agent – malaria, measles, tuberculosis, syphilis, and so on – were regarded as diseases by 95 per cent of laymen, and were regarded as diseases by 99 per cent of medical men. For both groups (lay and medical), the paradigm sort of disease was an infection – a condition was most likely to be classified as a disease if it was an infection. Of the conditions that were due to physical agents – drowning, tennis elbow, heat stroke, fractured skull and so on – 9 per cent of laymen regarded them as diseases, while 44 per cent of medical men classified them as diseases. Of the conditions that were due to chemical agents – barbiturate overdose, hangover, carbon-monoxide poisoning, lead poisoning, and so on – 16 per cent of laymen classified them as diseases, while 54 per cent of medical men thought that they were diseases (Campbell, Scadding and Roberts, 1979, pp.757–62).

This study illustrates a number of things. Firstly, that a distinction *is* drawn between pathological conditions regarded as diseases and those that are not. Secondly, this distinction is drawn by medical and laymen alike. And thirdly, that although there is a difference in the extensions of the lay and medical concepts – the medical concept of disease being more liberal – both are operating with recognizably the same concept of disease. We must now examine the nature of this distinction.

## Do diseases constitute a natural kind?

The question we need to answer here is whether all diseases share an explanatory nature which sets them apart from conditions which are not diseases. In order for diseases to constitute a (higher-order) natural kind, they must all have explanatory natures of a characteristic type not shared by other pathological conditions.

But diseases do not form a higher-order natural kind – being a disease does not consist in having a nature of a particular type. There are two arguments that show this. First, diseases in fact do not share a distinctive type of nature that marks them off as a distinct higher-order natural kind. Second, we know *a priori* that even if all diseases in fact shared a distinctive nature, this would still not show that being a disease consisted in having a particular nature.

Take the distinction between injury and disease – the natures of diseases are not of a different type from the natures of injuries. For example, if a man is savaged by a lion, we do not consider that he has acquired a disease – the process whereby he receives such characteristic injuries is not regarded as a disease. Similarly, if a man is devoured by killer ants, we still do not classify this biological interaction as a disease. However, the interaction with yet smaller organisms (like fungi, bacteria, or viruses), and the interaction with organisms that are not visible (like gastrointestinal worms) *are* considered to be diseases. Yet there do not seem to be any theoretically important differences between the extremes – all are interactions with other organisms where man is adversely affected, and just how big or visible the organism is seems theoretically unimportant. Just as each interaction with a small organism has its characteristic cluster of signs and symptoms, so too does the interaction with larger organisms leave its characteristic marks. The existence of a gradation of sizes of noxious organisms undermines the thesis that there is something special about the interaction with organisms of a minimal size – there is nothing special about the interaction with small or hidden organisms that marks them off as a natural kind.

Or take the injuries due to burns. If a baby burns himself in a fire, we consider that he has received an injury, and not acquired a disease. Similarly, if he is burnt by boiling water or hydrochloric acid, and receives similar burns, we do not think that he has undergone some disease process. Rather, he has been injured. On the other hand, suppose that the baby has a staphylococcal skin infection, and receives similar damage to the skin resulting in similar 'burns' – the clinical picture is so similar to burns that it has been called the 'Scalded Baby Syndrome'! In spite of the fact that the underlying inflammatory changes are similar, only in the latter case do we say the baby has a disease.

Similarly, there is no theoretically important difference between diseases and defects, disabilities, and deformities. For example, let us look at a genetic disease and a genetically determined disability. Phenylketonuria is a genetic disorder due to the absence of the enzyme phenylalanine hydroxylase, which leads to the accumulation of a toxic substance that produces the disability of mental retardation. Myopia is a genetically determined defect where the abnormal growth of the eye ball produces the disability of short-sightedness. There seems to be no theoretically important difference between these two processes that marks that one off as a disease and the other as not. Thus it seems that diseases do not fall into a distinct natural kind as opposed to defects, disabilities, and deformities.

Symptoms, signs, and syndromes also do not have distinctively different natures from diseases. For example, jaundice has a nature just as diseases have natures. Someone is jaundiced only if he has the explanatory nature of increased bilirubin in the tissues. The only difference between the class of jaundiced patients and those with some disease, for example, hepatitis B, is the order of the kind – the natural kind consisting of those patients that are jaundiced is a higher-order natural kind than the natural kind consisting of those patients with hepatitis B.

Similarly, there is nothing in the natures of syndromes like diabetes mellitus apart from their order that marks them off as being different from diseases. (Patients with diabetes mellitus constitute a natural kind – they all share the nature of impaired insulin functioning.) But this difference in order does not show that diseases have different kinds of natures. Diseases are not always the lowest order of natural kind either. Malaria is a disease entity, but can exist in a number of forms each of which constitutes a lower-order natural kind (each with a characteristic syndrome and nature). But the fact that malaria consists of a number of lower-order natural kinds (disease-form natural kinds) does not disqualify it from being a disease entity. Thus there is nothing in the nature of jaundice or diabetes mellitus that mark them off as non-diseases.

A similar argument can be constructed to show that the nature of diseases is not of a distinctively different sort from the nature of pathological states. Patients with cirrhosis of the liver have a cluster of signs and symptoms that is explained by a certain pathological state of the liver. Patients with hepatitis B too have a cluster of signs and symptoms which is explained by a certain interaction with a virus. There is a difference in the generality of the natures of these conditions, but this is not sufficient to enable us to mark off diseases as a distinct natural kind from pathological states or lesions.

Similarly, some cases of poisoning are classified as diseases, whereas others are not. For example, chronic lead-poisoning is classified as a disease. But barbiturate overdose is not. Yet there does not seem to be any theoretical property that the one nature has and the other lacks that makes the one a disease and the other not. Both are due to the interference in the normal functioning of the body by a chemical agent.

Finally, if we take a condition like starvation which is not classified as a disease, and a condition like kwashiorkor that is, we again do not find that the one has a nature that marks it off as a disease. Starvation is due to the deprivation of food, and kwashiorkor is a disease of children due to the deprivation of protein in the diet. They thus do not have a theoretically important difference between their natures.

So it seems that there is little reason to believe that diseases constitute a natural kind. In addition, if we look at the natures of all those conditions that we take to be diseases – for example, schizophrenia, malaria, syphilis, multiple sclerosis, motor-neurone disease, phenylketonuria, epilepsy, insulin-dependent diabetes, achondroplasia, and so on – they seem so diverse that it is difficult to see what property they all share in virtue of which they are the natures of diseases.

According to the second argument, even if it were the case that bodily conditions that we classified as diseases all shared a special sort of explanatory nature, this does not mean that being a disease consists in having a particular nature. Suppose we discovered that all diseases were due to fungal infections, and that other pathological conditions were due to bacterial infections. We know *a priori* that if we came across a condition that was due to a bacterial infection, but which consisted in our developing green spots, fever, malaise, and the complete failure of our blood to clot, it would be a disease. Because we know that it would be a disease *prior* to the discovery of its nature, being a disease cannot consist in membership to some higher-order natural kind – that is, it cannot consist in the possession of a special sort of nature. And hence diseases do not constitute a natural kind.

We can draw a number of conclusions from this. Firstly, because diseases do not constitute a natural kind, 'disease' does not have an NKS. If it did, we would have to conclude that there were no such things as diseases (because there was no such natural kind). But since we do not, 'disease' must have a descriptive meaning.

Secondly, we can no longer defend the idea that diseases-status is something that we discover. If all and only diseases shared a particular sort of explanatory nature, then the disease-status of some condition would be something that we could discover. We would discover this by seeing whether the condition fell into the same natural kind as such conditions as TB, lung cancer, etc. But since diseases do not constitute of a natural kind, the disease-status of some condition is not something that we can discover. It must instead be something that we invent. The line between diseases and other pathological conditions is not something that exists independently of us (and awaits discovery), but instead is something that we impose ourselves. Being a disease does not consist in having some special sort of nature.

## Do diseases have a nominal essence?

If diseases do not share a particular real essence in virtue of which they are all diseases, it is natural to ask whether diseases have a nominal essence. All diseases do seem to share some properties – all diseases are processes – they have an onset, a typical course, and an outcome. This is in contradistinction to certain of the other negative medical conditions like defects, deformities, disabilities, lesions, and injuries. If part of the nominal essence of disease is that diseases are processes that can evolve, this would explain just why it is that these other negative medical conditions are not classified as diseases. For these terms refer to static states of the body rather than processes. As Downie and Telfer put it:

> But it should be noticed that deformity, unlike illness and disease, is not *as such* incompatible with good health. Of course there are some deformities, such as 'a hole in the heart' which produces mechanical failures like those of illness, and a sufferer from these is said to be in poor health, as we say earlier. But a 'thalidomide baby' who has only vestigial limbs can still be described as *healthy*. Similarly, a child who is born with a malformation of the ears which makes him deaf is not called

71

unhealthy. It is true that a person who is severely handicapped in this way might hesitate before stating on a form that he is in good health, but broadly speaking these handicaps, severe though they are, are somehow not thought of as impairing health. ... The explanation seems to be that illness and disease are seen as things which essentially progress or change in a law-like manner, which have a life of their own. ... In such cases one can always sensibly ask whether the sufferer is getting better or worse. Being ill is essentially an *unstable* situation. The thalidomide victim, by contrast, is fixed in his disability, and so he is not regarded as unhealthy because there is nothing untoward *going on* in him (Downie and Telfer, 1980, p.20).

What is being suggested here is that if some condition is not a process, it is not a disease. Caroline Whitbeck agrees: 'Diseases, unlike injuries and impairments, are *processes*' (Whitbeck, 1978, p.210). Injuries might undergo changes – most injuries undergo a process of healing. But the fact that a skull fracture can be healed (and so have a natural history) does not mean that a skull fracture *is* a process.

A state is said to exist if and only if some particular (or set of particulars) has some property (or stand in some relation to one another) at a particular time. A process is said to exist if and only if some particular (or set of particulars) has a sequence of causally connected properties (or stand in a sequence of causally connected relations to one another) over a period of time. Thus processes necessarily take time, necessarily have a beginning and an end (if they are finite), and are the sort of thing that can get better or worse. While on the other hand, states do not necessarily take time, and do not have a beginning or end, and cannot have properties that imply that some change has been taking place – that is, they cannot get better or worse.

If we look at certain conditions, we can pick out those that are processes by seeing whether it makes sense to ask how long the condition takes, or when it began or ended, or whether it has become better or worse. Using these criteria, conditions like malaria and multiple sclerosis are obviously processes – they have a beginning, an end, they take time, and they can get better or worse. On the other hand, deformities like club foot and injuries like skull fracture do not take time – they are static states that exist at a time and do not need a period of time to exist. Admittedly one might ask how a fracture or deformity is 'coming along', but here one is talking not so much about these states but the *healing* of these states. It makes sense to ask how long the healing of a fracture took, and how the healing of the fracture is progressing, but it does not make sense to ask these same questions of the fracture itself. In order for us to make sense of questions of injuries and defects like 'How long did it take?', we have to expand the question into one like 'How long did it take *to acquire*, or *to heal?*' And therefore fractures and deformities are not processes. And if diseases are necessarily processes, they are not diseases.

However, being a process is not sufficient to differentiate diseases from all the other negative medical conditions (and normal conditions). Drowning, heat stroke, frostbite, and so on, all take time, but they are not diseases. Starvation and frostbite are the sort of conditions that have an onset, a course during which they can get better or worse, and an outcome. Thus we need a further characterization of disease processes to exclude those negative medical conditions that are processes but not diseases.

One thought is that diseased patients have something wrong with them, while those with injuries, or heatstroke, or overdoses, do not. But it is difficult to make sense of this idea. It is true that before being injured, or drowned, there is nothing wrong with the person. But once he acquires a fractured leg, for example, there is certainly something wrong with him – he has a leg that will not work properly. But the same is true with diseases – prior to becoming diseased, there need be nothing wrong with the person.

Perhaps the idea is that injuries, poisonings, and conditions like frostbite, sunburn, and so on, come from without – have external causes, while diseases come from within – they have internal causes. But the distinction between diseases and other pathological conditions cannot turn on this idea, because the source of infectious diseases is also external to the affected person.

There does not seem to be some property that diseases have and that other negative medical conditions lack. And if this is the case, then diseases do not even have a nominal essence: there is not a set of necessary and sufficient conditions for something to qualify as a disease rather than some other pathological condition. I may not have looked hard enough for such a definition, and there might be one that draws the boundaries between diseases and those we take just to be negative medical conditions, but it is difficult to see what it would be!

## Disease and explanation

There are two remaining questions that we have to answer. The first is whether there is a distinction at all between diseases and pathological conditions, or whether the putative distinction is based on a mistaken belief. And secondly, just why it is that we have the distinction in the first place.

On one theory, the distinction between diseases and non-diseases is based on a mistaken belief. Perhaps we believed that diseases fell into a natural kind, or had some special property in virtue of which they were diseases, and for this reason introduced the distinction. Now that we have discovered that they do not fall into a natural kind, and do not have some special feature, we should either abandon the distinction, or include injuries and other pathological conditions as diseases.

For example, in the Ptolemaic theory of the planetary motions, the earth was not classified as a planet. This was because celestial bodies were only classified as planets if they moved, and the earth was supposed to be the stationary centre of the universe. So a distinction was made between the earth and the (other) planets, based on the false belief that it was only the other planets that moved. When Copernicus realized that the earth moved, the distinction between the earth and the other planets (to the horror of the Church) was abandoned – it had been based on a false belief.

Some support for the idea that our distinction between disease and other pathological conditions is also based on a false belief comes from the fact that medical practitioners have a more liberal concept of disease than lay people – they have in part abandoned the distinction between diseases and other pathological conditions by broadening the concept of disease to include other pathological conditions. This could be explained by the fact that medical men have the additional knowledge that there is not some special difference between diseases and non-diseases, and have concluded that these non-diseases should be regarded as diseases. When they discovered that there was no fundamental theoretical difference between diseases and other pathological conditions, they broadened their concept of disease to include other pathological conditions as diseases.

We could further defend the idea that the distinction is based on a false belief by pointing out that our Western concept of disease might have been based on the Hippocratic theory of disease which *did* see all diseases as having some common nature. That is, all diseases were humoural imbalances. The body was seen as consisting of four humours – yellow bile, black bile, blood, and phlegm, and health consisted in the proper balance of these four humours. If anything upset the balance (for example, the climate), such that one humour predominated, the individual would acquire a disease. For example, in the winter months, the cold weather would influence the cold and watery humour (that is, phlegm) to predominate, thereby causing colds and bronchitis – the phlegm produced in these conditions was naturally evidence that there was an excess of phlegmy humour. All diseases on this theory, then, shared an identical nature – they all had the nature of having some humoural imbalance.

However, there are three reasons why this theory will not work. Firstly, medical men still preserve some distinction – starvation is still not considered a disease, and so on – and it is difficult to explain this if increased knowledge should lead to the abandonment of the distinction. If increased knowledge undermines a false belief that there is a fundamental theoretical difference between diseases and other pathological conditions, then we ought to abandon the distinction when we make the discovery. But we do not. Therefore, the distinction cannot be based on such a belief.

Secondly, the discovery that diseases do not have a nominal essence, or share a real essence in virtue of which they are diseases, does not incline us to suddenly regard drowning, or starvation, as a disease. And this is what we would expect if our distinction were to be based on a mistaken belief. Once we discovered that the distinction between the earth and the other planets was based on a mistaken belief, we abandoned the distinction. But we retain the distinction between diseases and other pathological conditions.

Thirdly, a great deal of historical evidence is needed to establish the thesis that the distinction is based on an old (now rejected) theory. The idea that the distinction is based on the Hippocratic theory of disease runs into difficulties over the supposed causes of personality. Hippocrates believed that differences in personality were due to minor excesses or humours. For example, a moody and melancholic (that is, black-biled) person was said to have a minor excess of black bile. But since this was not classified as a disease, Hippocrates himself did not believe that all and only all diseases shared a distinct nature (humoural imbalance) not shared by either normal conditions or other pathological conditions.

I think that the reason why we do not abandon our concept of disease when we discover that diseases do not share an underlying nature (real essence) or a set of superficial properties (nominal essence) is that our concept of disease is a family resemblance concept. Paradigm diseases like infections have an obscure onset, have a particular course, and have an outcome. They are conditions that evolve and have a characteristic natural history. Other conditions, like multiple sclerosis, are classified as diseases because they are much like infections – with an obscure cause, and course, and an outcome. Other conditions like injuries are less like these conditions because they have an obvious cause, and are not processes, even though the healing might take time. Again, drowning too has an obvious cause, and if it has a course at all, it is a very short one – paradigmatic diseases take longer to evolve. In this way, diseases can be shown to share a number of properties without there being any set that all and only diseases possess.

But we still face the question of why we have the distinction in the first place. Why draw a distinction between diseases and other negative medical conditions if no important difference is being picked out? We might begin to answer this question by noting that there *does* seem to be some property that all diseases have that non-diseases lack, and that is that diseases do not have obvious causes. (I mean 'easily observable' by 'obvious'.) Injuries, drownings, sunburn, barbiturate overdose, frostbite, starvation, and so on, all have obvious causes – that is, if we observed individuals acquiring these conditions, we would easily discern the cause of the condition. But not so for paradigmatic diseases – by observing people developing malaria, syphilis, multiple sclerosis – the cause is very obscure.

But this does not show that 'disease' *means* 'process with an obscure cause'. Jonathan Barnes points out that even in antiquity the cause of certain conditions, like rabies, was obvious, but rabies was nevertheless classified, and still is, as a disease (Jonathan Barnes in conversation). And even if we lived in a world where the causes of what we classify as disease were obvious, this would not mean that they would not be diseases. If malaria was caused by the bite of a mad cat, and multiple sclerosis was caused by the bite of a mad snake, and so on, the causes of these conditions would be obvious, but we would have no inclination to deny that they were diseases. So it seems that although diseases may have obscure causes, this is not something that is part of the meaning of the concept – the connection is purely contingent. However, it does remain a connection that demands explanation.

I think that the explanation of why we have the distinction between disease on the one hand, and those pathological conditions we do not take to be diseases on the other, lies in the origin of the concept. Robert Kendell puts it this way: 'Historically there can be little doubt that the concept of disease originated as an explanation for the onset of suffering and incapacity in the absence of obvious injury' (Kendell, 1975, p.10). The idea is that there was a need to explain suffering in the absence of an obvious cause. Because injuries had obvious causes, there was little need to develop a theory postulating something going on in the individual to explain his suffering. Whereas the same was not true of diseases – even cases like rabies needed the postulation of some on-going process to explain why a mad dog's bite led to anything more than just an injury.

This theory receives some support from pairs of similar conditions differently classified. For example, starvation is a condition brought about by lack of food and is not considered to be a disease. Whereas kwashiorkor is also a condition brought about by the lack of certain food (protein), but is considered to be a disease. This is, I think, best explained by the fact that the cause of kwashiorkor is not obvious – the children *do* get fed, it is just that the food is not of the correct sort, and this is not something that can be easily observed. And so the cause of kwashiorkor was obscure, and perhaps for this reason there was a need to postulate some on-going process in the children that could explain their condition. Similarly, the condition of chronic lead-poisoning did not have an obvious cause, and this seems to be the best explanation why it and not conditions like barbiturate overdose was classified as a disease.

The need for the postulation of some on-going process in some cases and not others led to the distinction between diseases and non-diseases. We have inherited the distinction, and preserve it because our concept of disease has become a family resemblance concept. We recognize now that injuries also stand in need of explanations. We think that barbiturate overdose, drunkenness, frostbite, and so on, also need the postulation of intervening processes (between obvious cause and resulting condition) if we are to explain the conditions. But we have inherited the historical division between diseases and other pathological conditions and continue to preserve it.

77

The conditions taken in the past to need an explanation might have received a similar sort of explanation at any one time, and this would have reinforced the distinction between diseases and non-diseases. Thus all obscurely caused conditions might initially have been explained by postulating the intervention by demons. This theory might later have been replaced by the theory that it was humoural imbalances that explained such obscurely caused conditions. More recently, the theory that all such conditions were due to infections by germs might have held sway. The fact that one theory was elaborated to explain such obscurely caused conditions may have fostered the grouping of such conditions together as diseases, and also fostered the Essentialist Fallacy.

The distinction might also have been preserved by the historical division between the professions of medicine and surgery. Perhaps it was those obvious injuries, like fractures, and frostbite, that constituted the domain of the surgeons who then treated them in a similarly obvious manner (by hacking off the offending parts, or splinting the crooked ones). On the other hand, the more sophisticated pathological conditions were handled by the physicians, who had to give fairly obscure remedies to match the obscurity of the cause of the conditions they were called upon to handle. The professional rivalry between physicians and surgeons might have led to physicians staking their claim to treat certain conditions. Perhaps their calling them diseases was a way of announcing to the surgeons that these conditions could only be treated by them, and was a way of warning them off.

Note that this can only be a theory of the *origin* of the distinction. This is because there are many conditions that fall under the surgeon's knife but which are nevertheless diseases. For example, appendicitis and breast cancer – not all conditions falling into the surgeon's domain are non-diseases. In any event, the issue of the origin of the distinction is something that we are going to have to leave to historians to discover.

In summary, diseases (as opposed to other pathological conditions) do not form a distinct natural kind. As well as not sharing a real essence in virtue of which all the conditions are diseases, diseases do not even have a nominal essence. Diseases might necessarily be processes, but we cannot give necessary and sufficient conditions for something to qualify as a disease as opposed to another pathological condition. This leaves us with the alternatives of giving up the distinction (because it is based on an error), or accepting that the concept of disease is a family resemblance concept. I have argued that we should adopt the latter view. Finally, I looked for an explanation why it is that those conditions we classify as diseases happen to have obscure causes (by and large), and why those conditions we classify merely as pathological conditions have obvious causes. The explanation lies in the origin of the concept of disease, as an intervening process need to explain suffering in the case of conditions that lacked an obvious cause. We have now inherited the distinction and preserve it because our concept is a family resemblance one. The explanation for the origin of the concept of disease is obviously an historical one, and one that must stand and fall on historical evidence.

We have examined the Essentialist Fallacy and seen that something is not a disease because it has a certain sort of nature. Nevertheless, the Essentialist Fallacy still continues to exert a powerful effect on our imagination. It has probably been entrenched into our thinking over history by our development of theories which explained all obscurely caused conditions in the same way.

# CHAPTER 5
# THE NORMAL AND THE PATHOLOGICAL

## Introduction

In Chapter 4 we saw that diseases do not constitute a higher-order natural kind. This means we have exposed the Essentialist Fallacy – some condition is not a disease in virtue of its nature. It also means that we cannot *discover* disease-status – the border between diseases and other pathological conditions does not exist independently of us and does not await discovery. Rather, it is a division that is invented by our adoption of one descriptive definition of disease rather than another. We could attribute a different meaning to the term 'disease' and thereby draw the boundary in a different place – it is up to us.

However, it is still possible that all pathological conditions share a distinctive type of nature different from normal conditions, and thereby constitute a distinct (higher-order) natural kind from normal conditions. If pathological conditions had a common type of explanatory nature not shared by normal conditions, then we could at least hope, by discovering what this general nature consisted in, to draw the line between normality and pathology in the right place. We could then have a means of discovering whether hyperactivity, or smoking, or stuttering, were pathological conditions, simply by discovering whether they possessed the right sort of explanatory nature.

What I will look at in this chapter is the question whether all pathological conditions constitute a natural kind – whether being pathological consists in having a particular nature. Again we encounter the Essentialist Fallacy. Here the fallacy consists in the belief that some condition is *pathological* because of the sort of nature that it has. If it turns out that pathological conditions do not share a real essence, I will explore the possibility that pathological conditions have a nominal essence.

80

### Do pathological conditions constitute a natural kind?

Do normal conditions fall into a higher-order natural kind that is distinct from the higher-order natural kind of pathological conditions? For these classes to constitute distinct natural kinds, the explanatory natures must fall into one of two distinct types. If this were the case, then by searching for the explanatory nature of a condition, we could discover whether the condition is part of normality or pathological. This would largely solve the problems we faced in the introduction.

For in some sense the solution to these problems does not turn so much on the discovery of the *disease* status of the borderline conditions, but on the discovery of the *pathological* status. This is because not a great deal turns on the decision about the disease status of a condition rather than, say, its injury status. For once we have decided on either status, we thereby decided that we ought to take steps to correct the condition, and that we ought to direct research to the discovery of the cure for it, that the NHS and insurance companies ought to cover the cost for its correction, and so on.

But pathological conditions do not constitute a natural kind. Firstly, the natures of pathological conditions do not in fact differ from the natures of non-pathological ones. For example, the nature of many plant diseases is characterized by the invasion of the plant by insects with the resultant damaging of the plant. Oak trees can become infested and damaged by the insect known as the oak-twig girdler. The female lays her eggs on new oak twigs, and when the eggs hatch the larvae bore into the twig in a spiral path causing the leaves behind the spiral to wither and die. Here we seem to have a pathological condition of an oak tree (Johnson and Lyon, 1976, p.210).

The mimosa tree also suffers from a condition that has much the same nature – the branches of the mimosa tree are destroyed by the insect known as the mimosa girdler. The female mimosa girdler lays her eggs in slits at the end of the branches of the mimosa tree. She then crawls back to the middle of the branches and gnaws a girdle around it – digging just deep enough to cut off the limb's circulation. The branch withers and dies, falls off the tree, scattering the beetle's eggs in the process (Batten, 1980, p.70).

In spite of the fact that this latter condition has a nature that closely resembles that of the oak tree's affliction, the 'infestation' of the mimosa tree is not pathological. It turns out that those trees that have the 'infestation' live twice as long as those without it. What the mimosa girdler is in fact doing is *pruning* the tree, and the tree is so far from being harmed by the process that it has evolved a special scent that attracts the mimosa girdler. Whether the condition is pathological or not does not seem to have anything to do with the nature of the condition, for in both cases we have a condition whose nature consists of the infestation by an insect with the subsequent destruction of branches by the interruption of the plant's circulation. The important thing is how the plant as a whole is affected by the condition (whatever its nature) – it is this that determines the pathological status of the nature, rather than the pathological status of the nature determining whether the condition counts as pathological.

Similarly, club-root disease of crucifers (cabbages and cauliflowers) is a fungal infectious disease of the roots that leads to stunting, yellowing, and wilting of the plants. In the cabbage, the fungus *Plasmodiophora brassicae* penetrates the root and enters into the individual cells, causing them to enlarge to form clubs. The fungus infested clubs utilize much of the food needed for the normal growth of the plant, and interfere with the absorption and transport of minerals and water through the roots, leading to stunting, yellowing, and wilting.

On the other hand, leguminous plants (for example, beans and peas) are infected by the bacterium *Rhizobium*. This bacterium penetrates the roots and enters into the individual cells, causing them to enlarge to ultimately form the root nodules. However, these nodules are essential for the well-being of the plant, for they enable the plant to fix nitrogen and to synthesize its own proteins. This almost identical process, far from being a disease as it was in the case of club-root disease, is a beneficial symbiosis (Agrios, 1978, p.501).

If we consult a standard text on plant pathology, we can see the Essentialist Fallacy at work. The authors argue that if a condition has the nature of a tumour (an abnormal proliferation of cells), it is *ipso facto* pathological. They write:

> Many terratomas [monstrously abnormal growths] such as
> nematode-induced root knots and Rhizobium-induced nodules
> are under the control of the pathogen [inducer of a
> pathological condition]. The structure and development of the

tumour are dictated by the pathogen for the benefit of the pathogen and when the needs of the pathogen are satisfied, the tumour stops growing. We say that these are self-limited terratomas. The host may benefit in the case of Rhizobium nodules or suffer in the case of nematode root knots (Horsfall and Couling, 1978, p.217).

The assumption here seems to be that it is because root nodules have the nature of a tumour that they are pathological (induced by pathogens). However, this is fallacious. It is not the case that the root nodule is pathological simply because it is a tumour – that is, because of its nature. It is not pathological because it is beneficial (and not harmful) to the plant.

There is a condition of apple trees known as the Hairy-Root Syndrome. This condition is due to the infection of roots by the bacterium *Agrobacterium rhizogenes*, producing fine hair-like projections on the roots. This condition is classified as a pathological condition because it causes stunting (Riker *et al.*, 1939, p.88). In other plants, fungal infection of the roots also leads to the production of fine rootlets. However, these fungal hyphae absorb nitrogen, phosphate and other nutrients more efficiently than the root hairs of uninfected plants, and thereby provide the plant with essential nutrients (Garrett, 1970, p.83). Here we have a condition with the same nature – infection of roots with the production of root-like projections – as the disease Hairy-Root Syndrome, but which is not itself pathological.

In a similar way, there are many conditions of man whose nature is characterized by their being infections by some micro-organism – for example, malaria, syphilis, leprosy, and so on. On the other hand, there are many other conditions of man that have the same explanatory nature – they are also infections, and yet they are not pathological conditions at all. For example, the colonization of the human infant's gastrointestinal tract by lactobacilli is something that benefits the infant – it protects him from the more pathogenic *Escherichia coli*. So it seems that being pathological does not consist in having a certain sort of explanatory nature.

The important point to take home from this example is that there are certain infections that we take to be diseases, and others that we take to be part of health. If we made the Essentialist Fallacy, we would treat our bowel flora with antibiotics, thereby giving ourselves a permanent low-grade diarrhoea. Since we would be free of an infection, we would conclude that we were free of some pathological condition. But this is absurd – nobody would see such a permanent low-grade diarrhoea as an improvement in health.

It might be suggested that pathological conditions *do* have a nature in virtue of which they are pathological – namely, they all have natures with the property of producing harm or malfunctioning. We simply beg the question that they have no common nature by excluding such a characterization from the outset. But in looking for a particular type of explanatory nature that makes a condition pathological, we have to find a feature of the nature of conditions that causally explains the relevant manifesting features. But to describe a nature as 'harmful' or 'productive of a malfunction' is to describe it in terms of its effects. But if we do this, then the nature can hardly to said to *explain* those effects. It seems then that if the nature of pathological conditions is to be explanatory and hence qualify as uniting the conditions into a single natural kind, it cannot consist of the property of having those effects it is supposed to explain. And therefore having the 'nature' of causing harm or malfunctioning does not qualify.

We also know *a priori* that pathological conditions do not constitute a natural kind. Suppose that we discover that all pathological conditions shared a similar nature – they were all cancers with a nature consisting of a mechanism producing cell division. We can imagine discovering that the continual division of cells that line the gastrointestinal tract (which is necessary to replace the loss of cells due to sloughage as food passes down the tract) has the same nature as any cancerous division of cells. The fact that the division of cells in the gastrointestinal tract had the same nature as a pathological condition would not make it pathological. Hence being pathological does not consist in having a particular essence.

Or suppose we discover that all pathological conditions are infections. We can still imagine discovering that the normal protection of our gastrointestinal tract from various pathogens has the same nature – that is, consists in the infection of our gastrointestinal tracts by protective flora. But this would not mean that this counts as a pathological condition. And so something is not pathological simply because of its membership to some particular natural kind.

There is a third argument that shows that pathological conditions do not form a natural kind. If certain types of processes were normal, they would not be classified as pathological – it is not their nature being of a certain type that makes them pathological, but their being abnormal that makes them so. Ageing is a process that involves many degenerative changes that harm the individual, gradually leading to death. Yet ageing is not classified as a disease. This is because the ageing process is normal.

Suppose that we normally lived to 200-years-old, then our present ageing process would represent an abnormal condition (we would regard it as a less malignant form of Progeria, perhaps calling it 'Ageria'). Even though ageria would have the same nature as ageing does now, it would be pathological because of its relation to the (new) norm. So it seems that it is the relation to the norm that makes a condition pathological, rather than the sort of nature that it has.

Fourthly, whether a process is pathological or not depends not just on its nature, but on the relation of the organism to the environment in which it lives – 'one environment's adaptation is another's disease'. For example, let us take sickle-cell trait. This is the trait of having an abnormal haemoglobin molecule that enables red cells to resist malarial parasites. Such a trait is obviously to the advantage of the host in an environment where malaria is endemic. But in environments of low oxygen concentration, such a trait leads to sickle-cell anaemia – the red cells become sickle-shaped, and rupture, leaving the person anaemic. Thus at high altitudes, sickle-cell trait would be a pathological condition. Whether it is pathological or not does not depend on its nature, but on the relation of the organism to the environment.

Similarly, on the mainland it is advantageous for flies to have wings that enable them to fly. But on islands with strong cross winds, it is disadvantageous to have wings that 'function' – for then the flies are swept out to sea and die. On the mainland, any genetic abnormality producing malformed wings is a pathological condition, while on the islands, the reverse is true – the island flies have in fact evolved 'malformed' wings (by mainlander standards) to have the function of preventing flies from being swept out to sea. Whether malformed wings are pathological depends in part on the relation of the fly to its environment, and not on the nature of the condition itself.

The pygmy people have an insensitivity to growth hormone. Let us assume that this trait enables them to hide from their prey amongst shrubs. Lacking such a sensitivity would be pathological among pygmies, while if the Masai were to acquire such an insensitivity in their environment, they would be classified as diseased – they are tall in order to facilitate cooling, and would probably suffer in their environment if they were short like the pygmy. Whether a condition is pathological does not depend just on its type of nature. It depends crucially on the relation of the organism to the environment.

Similarly, in an environment with our western habit of overeating, the predisposition to acquire diabetes is classified as a pathological defect. Indians are known to have a much greater incidence of diabetes than their western counterparts. Many have wondered whether there is some environment where the predisposition is not a defect. In 1979, Douglas Coleman experimented with normal mice and mice with a genetic suscept-ibility to diabetes. He fed them as much food and water as they wanted, and after one week he cut off all food supply, while preserving their access to water. The results were startling – the mice susceptible to diabetes lived up to 46 per cent longer than the normal mice. The susceptibility seems to enable the mice to survive in times of famine (Harsanyi and Hutton, 1983, p.128). This seems to be the reason why the trait is so common among Indians who have experienced many food shortages. It seems that the trait can be a defect in one environment (where food is plentiful), while it can be an advantage in another (where food may often be scarce).

In fact, for any genetic disorder we like, we can imagine an environment where it would *not* be pathological. For example, hereditary deafness would be an advantage in a world filled with very loud and disturbing noise. Albinism – the failure to produce the pigment melanin – is a pathological condition because it fails to prevent damage of the skin from the sun's rays. However, if the amount of light in our world were greatly reduced (in a nuclear freeze), it would be an advantage because it would enable the skin to synthesize vitamin D from the small amount of light available. (It is well known that blacks living outside the tropics are susceptible to rickets and osteomalacia because their pigmented skin prevents the synthesis of vitamin D. This is presumably why caucasians became white.)

There is a final argument that shows that pathological conditions do not constitute a natural kind distinct from normal conditions. We argued above that any natural kind must have a distinct explanatory nature – without natural divisions existing among the natures of the different natural kinds, no sense can be made of the idea that the divisions among objects exist independently of us, and are therefore discovered and not invented. Now there is reason to suspect that some pathological conditions have a nature that is neither qualitatively distinct from nor quantitatively discontinuous with the nature of normality. Some diseases seem to vary only in degree from the norm. As George Pickering comments about hypertension:

> The conviction is steadily growing that there is no natural dividing line between normal blood pressure and hypertension, and to create one is to create an artifact. . . . Essential hypertension seems to be a disease of a different kind in which the fault is not of kind but of degree; the deviation is not qualitative but quantitative (Pickering, 1962, p.87).

If hypertension is a pathological condition, but nevertheless has a nature that differs only in degree from the norm, with intermediates occurring between the extremes, then pathological conditions cannot constitute a distinct natural kind from normal conditions, for we have at least one pathological condition that is not a distinct natural kind from normality.

There is a possibility that all diseases turn out to be deviations in degree from the norm. For example, the nature of diabetes may consist simply in the production of less insulin than normal. That there appears to be a discontinuity between diabetics and normal individuals is due to the 'threshold effect' – only at a certain concentration of blood glucose will the kidney fail to reabsorb it all, and so only at this level will glucose spill over into the urine causing polyuria, polydipsia, and glycosuria (Lewontin, 1982, p.54). If this is so, then pathological conditionss do not constitute a distinct natural kind – the pathological status of the condition does not depend on its having a certain explanatory nature, but on its being abnormal.

Thus pathological conditions do not constitute a natural kind. A condition is not pathological because of its type of nature, but because of its effect on the organism and because of its deviation from the norm.

This has a number of important consequences. Firstly, it means that 'pathology' does not have an NKS. If it did and purported to refer to a natural kind, we would have to conclude that there were no pathological conditions because there is no such natural kind.

But this is absurd. Therefore it has a descriptive sense.

Secondly, we have exposed the Essentialist Fallacy – a condition is not pathological because it happens to have a particular sort of nature. Otherwise the protective colonization of our gastro-intestinal tract would be pathological.

Thirdly, this all means that we do not discover the pathological status of a condition. There is no discoverable natural boundary among conditions separating normal conditions from pathological ones. The line between these conditions is something we impose on the world by adopting one definition of the pathological rather than another.

Finally, we do not have an easy solution to the problems that we were faced with initially. We cannot settle, for example, the issue of whether we should treat over-active children by trying to discover whether hyperactivity falls into the natural kind of pathological conditions – there is no such kind.

## The nominal essence of pathology

In spite of these arguments, many still commit the Essentialist Fallacy. They assume that the pathological status of a condition depends on its type of nature. Bieber *et al.* in their book *Homosexuality: A Psychoanalytic Study*, seem to argue that homo-sexuality is a pathological condition because it is the result of a pathological relationship between the mother and son. The tacit assumption seems to be that the pathological status of homosexuality depends on the pathological nature of the relation-ship of mother and son. But Davison correctly points out that this merely begs the question: The intimate mother–son relationship is only pathological if one has already decided to classify homo-sexuality as a disease. He writes:

> Does the finding that male homosexuals have similar child-rearing experiences different from male heterosexuals demonstrate pathology? My answer is No. One cannot attach a pathogenic label to a pattern of child rearing unless one *a priori* labels the adult behaviour pattern as pathological. For example, Bieber *et al.* found that what they called a "close-binding intimate mother" was present much more often in the life histories of the analytic male homosexual patients than

among heterosexual controls. My question is simple. What is wrong with such a mother unless you happen to find her in the background of people whose current behaviour you judge beforehand to be pathological (Davison, 1976, p.159)?

He continues:

> Suppose we found that women who are now good golfers had as children attended public schools more often than did women who are poor golfers. Suppose also that the difference in their golfing ability is the only consistent one between the two groups. Under what circumstances would we conclude that childhood experiences in private schools are pathogenic, causing pathology or illness? The answer is simple: going to private school is pathogenic if its outcome, being a poor golfer, has already been judged pathological. If we do not make this *a priori* judgment, we cannot talk of a difference between two groups indicative of pathology in one of the group, and we cannot regard the presumed cause a pathogenic one. The most we can say is that the two groups are *different* from each other (Davison & Neale, 1978, p.315).

This argument might appear too swift. If we discovered that homosexuality was due to a viral infection, or a slow growing tumour of the 'sex orientation centre', would we not regard this as a discovery that homosexuality was a disease after all? And this *because* of the sort of nature that the condition has? But this is mistaken – we only *think* this would make it so because we feel that certain natures are intrinsically pathological. But I have shown that there is nothing in the nature of the process independently of its relation to some norm and its effect on the organism as a whole that makes the condition pathological.

Suppose we discovered that Einstein (and other geniuses) owed their intelligence to a unique intracerebral viral infection. In such a circumstance we would not look upon this infection as a disease, but as a *symbiotic* relationship. The infection would be something we would foster, and not 'cure'. In fact, it has been discovered that Einstein's brain contained an abnormal number of glial cells. Supposing that this was responsible for his genius, we will not find the condition in any pathological textbook. The pathological status of a condition does not derive from the type of nature that it has, but from its effects on the organism, and on the relation of the condition to the norm. There is no such thing as an intrinsically pathological nature.

Nevertheless, suppose we are wondering whether schizophrenia is a disease. Suppose we have a full characterization of the neurophysiological mechanisms that underly play-acting. Suppose too that we discover that these very same neurophysiological mechanisms are in operation in schizophrenics – we discover that their madness is all method. Then I think we would be inclined to think that schizophrenia is not a disease. And this *because* it was not caused by an abnormal process.

Such a view of schizophrenia has been put forward by Ronald Laing. He has argued that schizophrenia is not a disease because it is the product of the normal processes of strategy formation: 'The experience and behaviour that gets labelled schizophrenic is a specific strategy that a person invents in order to live in an unlivable situation' (Laing, 1967, p.78). Whether he is right about schizophrenia, it does seem correct to infer the non-pathological status of the condition from the normality of the underlying process. If such a process were considered a disease-process, we would have to consider *all* intentional behaviour as pathological. But this would be absurd. Hence, being an abnormal process is necessary for something to be pathological.

Pregnancy, menstruation, and teething result in significant discomfort and disability, but we do not regard them as pathological conditions because we take the processes that cause them to be normal. It is only if the underlying process is abnormal that we consider the condition to be pathological.

Thomas Szasz makes this point in discussing alcoholism, which he thinks is not a disease because it is the product of the normal processes of habit formation:

> Drinking to excess may cause illness, but in itself is not a disease – in the ordinary sense of the word 'disease'. Excessive drinking is a habit. According to the person's values, he may consider it a good or bad habit. If we choose to call bad habits 'diseases', there is no limit to what we may define as 'diseases' – and 'treat' involuntarily. The misuse of alcohol – whatever the reason for it – is no more an illness than is the misuse of any other product of human inventiveness, from language to nuclear energy (Szasz, 1972, p.84).

Alcoholism may resemble other pathological conditions, but if the process producing it, that is, its nature, is a normal one, then the condition (in spite of this resemblance) is not pathological.

The position here is different from the one that holds that pathological conditions constitute a natural kind. We know that pathological conditions do not have a distinctive type of explanatory nature. What is being claimed here is that in order to count as pathological a condition must have a nature that is of a type that is abnormal (and not that this nature be of a specific type).

Thus the discovery of the nature of a condition is in some way relevant to the classification of that condition as pathological. For example, suppose that we found that hyperactive children produced abnormally high quantities of certain neurotransmitters. Suppose too that putting such children on special diets reversed their hyperactivity. Are we not more justified here in regarding hyperactivity as a disease than if were to discover it was a manifestation of a (normal) desire to get attention?

The abnormality of the underlying process is necessary for the condition to be pathological, but it is not sufficient. We first have to conclude that hyperactivity is something that is doing the children harm, or resulting in some malfunction. If we have not already decided that it is harmful for children to be over-active (for whatever reason), we cannot argue from the fact that the underlying process is abnormal to the conclusion that the condition is pathological. We might find that all Russian dissidents have an excess of a certain neurotransmitter and are sensitive to a certain diet – if put on a special diet (of bread and water!), they cease to cause trouble for the Soviet authorities. This discovery however would not constitute conclusive evidence that dissidence is a disease!

The question 'Do pathological conditions have a nominal essence?' can now be answered in part. Let us put forward this tentative definition:

Some condition is pathological if and only if it has an explanatory nature that is of a type that is abnormal and that causes harm or malfunctioning.

This definition is not very revealing because we have not given any account of what it is to be abnormal, and because we have not decided whether being pathological is related to harm or to malfunctioning. In Chapters 6 to 9 I will be examining whether the connection is to the notion of harm or to the notion of malfunctioning. I will now look at the notion of abnormality.

## The nature of norms of health

There are three concepts of the normal and the abnormal that offer themselves as candidates for use in the definition of disease and pathology. The first concept I will call the 'Empirical' concept. The norm for a particular class of objects with respect to a particular property is determined in an empirical way by discovering what the mean for that property is, and seeing what falls within two standard deviations of that mean. What falls outside this range is abnormal. This is what Peter Alexander calls the 'statistical concept':

> If we take a normal curve and mark off a central portion of it where by far the greatest number of individuals fall [95% if we take two standard deviations] and designate those individuals 'normal', we are using the statistical concept of normality. It is just a matter of fact if some feature of the world conforms to this pattern. To say that x is normal, in this sense, is just to say that it is, in some respect, as x's usually are (Alexander, 1973, p.139).

The problem is that if we define the pathological in terms of this norm, it will either be unacceptable or circular. It will be unacceptable if the norm is derived from a population that is not (by and large) pathology-free. Any widely shared pathological condition will then not count as abnormal, and hence not be pathological. For example, dental caries is a disease that practically every Westerner suffers from – it is not an unusual condition. Nevertheless, it is pathological. But if being abnormal is a necessary condition for being pathological, then we cannot say that dental caries is a pathological condition.

It has now become evident that the Japanese are short not because of any racial characteristics, but because of poor nutrition. It has been discovered that Japanese brought up on an American diet are significantly taller than their Japanese counterparts, and are no longer shorter than the Americans. We want to be able to conclude that most Japanese are suffering from (mild) malnutrition. However, if we use the Empirical norm, we are precluded from recognizing anything pathological about their being short. Because it is average, we have to conclude that it is not pathological.

In the past, whole communities suffered from a single infectious disease – malaria was so common in the Upper Mississippi Valley during the early nineteenth century that its manifestations were regarded as normal, but it was still a disease (Wing, 1978, p.19). Dyschromic spirochaetosis, the spirochaetal infectious disease with significant mortality and morbidity, is so common in a South American tribe that those who lack it are regarded as abnormal and excluded from marriage. But it is still a disease (Dubos, 1965, p.251). Amongst many African tribes, intestinal worms is so common that people regard them as part of normality. But in spite of the fact that these conditions are normal (in the sense of being average), they are still diseases.

In addition, on this account of the norm, we preclude ourselves from discovering that we are all suffering from some as yet unrecognized disease. Perhaps we all accumulate minute amounts of copper in our brains and this lowers our IQ by 30 points. We want to be able to say that this is a pathological condition, but this is precluded if we adopt the empirical concept. We do not want to claim merely that such a condition can *become* pathological or a disease when we have 'cured' most people of it! We want to be able to say that it is *now* a pathological condition.

It is not only acquired diseases/pathology that we are precluded from recognizing. Suppose that originally we all lived to 200-years-old. Just as some people now suffer from progeria (premature ageing), imagine there were some individuals in our evolutionary past who suffered from a less malignant form called 'Ageria' that ended their lives at 70-years-old. Suppose a catastrophe happend to kill all those who did not have ageria. Then we would all come to suffer from a hereditary disease. Compare the case where a nuclear holocaust kills all of us except those suffering in a remote clinic from Huntington's chorea. Would not all humans come to suffer from this hereditary disease?

On the other hand, if we derive the norm from a population that we have first determined is pathology-free, the account will be circular. We need to exclude diseased individuals in order to determine the reference population and the (correct) norm, but we need the norm to determine which are the diseased individuals. And so pathology and disease cannot be defined in terms of the empirical norm.

The second concept of the norm is what I will call the 'Idealized' concept. Here the norm is not determined by some empirical statistical method. Although we are influenced by what is usual, we decide upon the norm because of the consequences that such a norm generates. If the norm generates unacceptable consequences – for example, that dental caries is not a disease, or that all intentional action is the product of a disease – then we reject that particular norm, and select one with more acceptable consequences. On this concept, we decide that alcoholism is not pathological when we find out it is simply a bad habit, because to conclude it is pathological would mean that all habits were diseases. In this way, we are not faced with the vicious circle undermining the Empirical concept.

Adopting one norm rather than another has the practical consequence of making us concentrate on the cure of those conditions that turn out to be pathological. By drawing the norm in one place, we are in effect saying that we ought to cure these conditions first before we concentrate on those normal conditions like ageing that we would all be better off without.

We choose one norm rather than another because we wish to create certain priorities in dealing with all those conditions that we would be better off without. We would all be better off if we did not age, if we did not suffer from a need to sleep for 8 hours a day, if we did not synthesize uric acid and thereby be liable to gout, etc. But we are not diseased because of this – we are not diseased because we are not supermen! On the other hand, we would be better off without dental caries, but we regard it as an abnormal process because we choose to give its cure the same priority as we give to the cure of TB and multiple sclerosis. And so we regard it as a disease. We regard the process of ageing as normal, because we consider that it is more important first to rid ourselves of those processes we take to be abnormal. On the other hand, if it became as important to us to reverse the ageing process as it was to reverse cancer, we *would* come to think of ageing as an abnormal process, and classify it as a pathological condition. The content of the second account of a norm is given by its practical consequences.

The last account of the norm I will call the 'Theoretical' concept. Here the content of the norm is not given by its practical or normative consequences, but by its theoretical consequences. Anthony Flew argues that using a norm to define disease does not imply that the concept will be a normative one:

Consider, for example, the status of the First Law of Motion in classical mechanics or the Principle of Population in the theoretical scheme or Thomas Robert Malthus. Both lay down ideal norms, all deviations from which have to be explained: explained by reference to 'impressed forces' in the former case; and in the later by the operation of various 'positive and preventative checks'. But no one (one hopes) is rooting: either for the removal of all impressing forces; or for the liquidation of all checks on population growth. . . . It is in the same way possible to develop a completely detached, objective, non-prescriptive ideal norm of health; an ideal norm defined in terms of the fulfilling of the function which organs and organisms appear to have, yet have not, been designed to fulfil (Flew, 1983, p.109).

However, if the content of the norm is theoretical, then there must presumably be some way of learning that any 'objective' norm corresponds to reality. But I have argued that there *is* no natural boundary to be discovered between normal and pathological conditions, and hence the norm cannot be theoretical. The only content that can be given is in terms of the *consequences* that the norm carries, that is, in its prescriptive content.

It might be argued that a theoretical norm need not correspond to anything in reality. Take the theoretical norm that bodies continue in their state of rest of rectilinear uniform motion unless disturbed by a force. Conventionalists argue that there are no such things in the universe as forces, and hence that this norm does not correspond to anything in reality. A force is defined in terms of what motion is considered 'natural', that is, not requiring any force for its maintenance. What motion is taken as natural is up to us. Aristotle defined rest as natural motion, and forces were required to sustain objects in uniform motion. This theory meant that the laws of motion became somewhat complicated. Galileo's theory that uniform circular motion or rest was natural was more attractive because the laws of motion became much more simplified. Finally, Newton's theory that rectilinear uniform motion or rest was natural is even more attractive. It made the laws of motion much simpler again. Nevertheless, one could still argue that there are no such things as forces in the world, and that norms of motion are chosen to simplify records of motion. One could argue that Newton's theory was accepted not because it was more accurate, but because it was a simpler summary.

If we take this view of theoretical norms, we can show that norms need not be prescriptive – the First Law of Motion is hardly prescriptive! But then the norm is hardly 'objective' either. More importantly, since the simplicity of expressing laws of nature does not enter into the health issue, it is difficult to see what content (besides the prescriptive one) can be given to the norm.

The criterion of choosing the norm that generates the simplest theory is not used when we come to select the norms of health. Even if it were simpler to regard the colonization of our gastrointestinal tracts as a disease (because it shares the same nature with other pathological conditions such as infections), this would not mean that it is after all pathological! Even if it is simpler to regard the degenerative diseases as part of health (because they share the same nature as normal degeneration through ageing), this would not mean that they are part of health! Thus we cannot argue that the norms of health have any theoretical content.

Let me illustrate how the prescriptive content of the norm might influence the classification of the condition as pathological. George Engel argues that grief is a disease:

> [A]s with classic diseases, ordinary grief constitutes a distinct
> syndrome with a relatively predictable symptomatology which
> includes, incidentally, both bodily and psychological
> disturbances. It displays the autonomy typical of disease; that
> is, it runs its course despite the sufferer's efforts or wish to
> bring it to a close. A consistent aetiologic factor can be
> identified, namely, a significant loss (Engel, 1961, p.18).

It would be a mistake (noted above) to argue that because it is normal (in the empirical sense) to respond to emotional loss with grief, grief is not a disease. It is normal (in this sense) to respond with measles and mumps to the appropriate virus, but this does not mean that they are not diseases.

With the Idealized norm, we could construct a norm in terms of which (appropriate) grief was a pathological condition. But this has undesirable consequences – we want to be the sort of people in whom it is healthy to respond to loss with grief, and so we do not want to adopt a norm with the consequence that grieving becomes a disease, and something we should cure with drugs. For this reason, then, we adopt one norm rather than another.

An important factor that will influence whether to regard some process as normal is the ability we have to treat the condition medically. We are unlikely to regard ageing as a disease, even though we would be better off without it, because we are at present unable to do anything about it. However, if we discovered a drug that enabled us to live healthy lives to 200-years-old, would we not come to view the drug as vitamin F, and regard our present ageing process as abnormal and as a vitamin-deficiency disease? As Joseph Margolis remarks:

> Imagine, for instance, that an extraordinary discovery confirms that a certain drug could increase our life expectancy, fourfold: that it would be inexpensive, accessible, and without unfavourable side effects: *and* that society would begin to adjust its expectations and social arrangements to the increased longevity of its members. Might not patterns of now-normal decline leading to eventual death 'by natural causes' come to be viewed as disease syndromes, severely dysfunctional processes subject to medical correction? If not, why not (Margolis, 1976, p.89)?

Thus, a process or condition must be of a type that is abnormal in the idealized sense if it is to be pathological. This norm is selected because of its practical consequences. That is, it has a prescriptive content. Pathological conditions do not constitute a natural kind with a distinctive sort of explanatory nature that marks them off from normal conditions. A condition is pathological if and only if it has a nature of a type that is abnormal and that produces harm or malfunctioning.

I have exposed the Essentialist Fallacy – being pathological does not consist in having a particular nature. This has grave consequences for our problem of classification. We cannot solve the problem of whether smoking, or hyperactivity, or stuttering are pathological by simply uncovering their natures – they are not pathological in virtue of the nature that they have. Rather, they are pathological if their nature is abnormal and if this nature gives rise to either harm or malfunctioning. The task immediately ahead is to discover whether disease and pathology is connected to the property of harm or the property of malfunctioning, and whether these concepts are value-laden.

# CHAPTER 6
# THE CONCEPT OF FUNCTION

## Introduction

A definition of disease in terms of the concept of function is attractive. On such a definition the issue of whether some condition is or is not a disease is a matter of objective fact. It is a matter of objective fact because whether something is a disease will depend on the way the world is, and not on such subjective factors as personal values, preferences, or decisions. Once different people have understood the concept, it will be the facts and not our fiats that determine what are diseases.

With such a definition, agreement can be achieved in disputes over disease-status, and mistakes exposed. Once everyone is in possession of all the objective facts, they will agree as to what are and are not diseases, and we will be able to expose certain factual mistakes. We can show that the South American Indians are mistaken to think that dyschromic spirochaetosis is not a disease because it produces a malfunction. Similarly, we can show that Samuel Cartwright was mistaken to think that runaway slaves had the disease drapetomania.

It will also be possible, by accumulating more biological facts, for us to settle the debates over whether the NHS ought to pay for Nicorette, or whether the insurance companies should pay for the treatment of stuttering, and so on. All we need to do is to discover the facts about our functional capacities.

In addition, with such a definition we can justify our criticism of those who make mistaken disease attributions. If disease was defined in terms of subjective matters like (personal) values, then it would be legitimate for those with different values to classify conditions differently. And we could not justify our criticism of their deviant classification. For example, we could not justifiably criticize Russian psychiatry for classifying dissidence as a disease.

98

But on an objective definition of disease, such a criticism would be justified.

There are thus many attractions to having an objective concept of disease. However, an account of disease in terms of the concept of malfunctioning will only be an objective and value-free account if the concept of function is itself objective and value-free. Hence we need to examine the concept of function.

I have argued that pathological conditions (of which diseases are one sort) can be understood in terms of conditions with a nature of a type that is abnormal and that leads to harm or malfunctioning. The issue remains whether the connection is to the notion of harm, or whether to the notion of malfunction, and this is what Chapters 6 to 9 will determine.

The analysis of the concept of function is also needed to settle the Naturalist–Normativist debate as to whether the concept of disease is value-laden or not. Naturalists hold that the concept of disease is to be understood in terms of the concept of malfunction, and that this is a value-free account of the concept because the concept of function (and malfunction) is value-free. On the other hand, the Normativists hold that the concept of disease is to be understood in terms of the concept of harm, and that this is a value-laden account because the concept of harm is value-laden.

Diseases will obviously be the malfunctionings of biological parts. But there are not two different concepts of function here – one for biological parts and one for artefacts – a biological part has a function in essentially the same way that the part of an artefact has a function – the mammalian heart has a function in the same way that spark-plugs have a function. The best explanation of why we use the same word in these contexts is that we mean the same thing in both cases. I will examine three rival theories of the concept of function, but before this I will explore some philosophic problems that we would like our analysis of the notion of function to solve.

## The problems

A good analysis of function should provide solutions to the following philosophic problems. As Andrew Woodfield puts them:

(1)  Hempel's problem. Why is it that only some of an item's

activities are functions, and the others are accidental?
(2) Nagel's problem. Why is it that we ascribe functions to the parts of some systems (like organisms) but not to the parts of others (like the solar system)?
(3) The problem of functional explanation. How can it be explanatory of an item to cite one of its effects? (Woodfield, 1976, p.108).

Let us examine these problems briefly in turn.

Firstly, we make a distinction between effects that are accidents and those that are functions. Our noses have many effects, but only some are its functions: it has the function of heating and humidifying inspired air, but it is just a happy accident that it has the effect of supporting spectacles. As Larry Wright argues:

> If a small nut were to work itself loose and fall under a value-adjustment screw in such a way as to adjust properly a poorly adjusted valve, it would make an accidental contribution to the smooth running of the engine. We would never call the maintainence of proper value adjustment the *function* of the nut. If it got the adjustment right, it was just an accident (Wright, 1973, p.151).

Thus we make a distinction between accidental effects and the function of a part, and we would want our concept of function to preserve this distinction.

Secondly, only certain systems have parts with functions. Organisms have parts with functions, but the solar system does not. Just as the parts of an organism do whatever is needed to serve the goals of survival and reproduction, so the parts of the solar system do whatever is needed to keep the total sum of kinetic and potential energy constant. But we do not consider that some planetary motion has the function of keeping this quantity constant, while we do consider that the heart has the function of serving the goals of survival and reproduction. Not every seemingly goal-directed system has parts which serve various functions. Thus we make a distinction between such systems, and we want our concept of function to preserve the difference between the effects of parts in such systems.

Thirdly, citing the function of a part can explain why that part occurs in some system. 'Why do mammals have hearts?' can be correctly answered by 'because they have the function of pumping blood'. The explanatory power of functions is closely related to the distinction between accidents and functions: the existence of the nose is explained by its function of heating and humidifying inspired air, but it is not explained by its happening to support spectacles. Larry Wright gives this example:

> 'What is the function of the vinyl cover on the playing field?' and 'Why is there a vinyl cover on the playing field?' both demand the same answer here: to keep the rain off. The ascription of a function simply *is* the answer to a 'Why?' question, and one with etiological force. If 'to keep the rain off' does not account for the cover's being there, if it is just something the cover is good for, like making puddles for the kids to play in, then it does not give the cover's function; neither does it answer the 'Why?' question (Wright, 1976, p. 80).

Thus we can see that the ascription of a function to a part can explain why that part is there, and we want our concept of function to explain how this ascription can be explanatory, while the ascription of an accident is not.

Now to the different theories of function.

## The evaluative theory

I will call any account of function an Evaluative Theory if it makes an irreducible reference to the good of the system. Such an account will have the following structure:

> The function of X (in Y) is Z if and only if (a) X does Z, and (b) X's doing Z contributes to the good of Y.

For example, John Canfield gives an Evaluative account of the concept of function:

> A function of I (in S) is to do C *means* I does C and that C is done is useful to S. For example '(In vertebrates) a function of the liver is to secrete bile' means 'The liver secretes bile, and that bile is secreted in vertebrates is useful to them' (Canfield, 1963, p.290).

Similarly, Richard Sorabji argues that there is one necessary condition for the concept of function:

> The condition is that the performance by a thing of its (putative) function should confer some *good*. This condition is met in our example concerning the function of the heart, for the circulation of blood does confer a good in that it promotes life (Sorabji, 1964, p.291).

However, the Evaluative Theory is mistaken: it cannot provide necessary or sufficient conditions for having a function, nor can it solve the philosophical problems about functions. Firstly, it cannot provide sufficient conditions for something to have a function. My nose may contribute to my good by supporting my spectacles, but this is not one of its functions. The production of heart sounds may aid diagnosis, and thereby serve the good of the individual, but this is not a function of the heart. The Duypetrens contracture on my hand may enable me to hang from a cliff edge and thereby save my life in some emergency, but this does not ensure it has a function.

Secondly, the Evaluative Theory cannot provide necessary conditions for having a function. To see this, it is necessary to understand that natural selection does not only lead to the evolution of traits that enhance the survival of the individual organism. Sexual selection can lead to the selection of traits that impair the survival chances of the individual, but which enhance the survival of such traits in the next generation. For example, the plumage of peacocks impairs the survival chances of each peacock, because it makes them more conspicuous to predators. However, the trait is selected because females find it attractive, and so males with the trait leave more offspring in the next generation.

Similarly, kin selection can lead to the selection of traits that impair the survival chances of the individual, but which nevertheless enhance the survival of such traits in the next generation. For example, the warning calls of Belding's ground squirrels impair the survival chances of the caller because they make the caller more conspicuous to predators. However, the trait is selected because by warning kin, who possess the same trait, it enhances their survival chances (and the survival of that trait in the next generation). Squirrels not possessing the trait are less likely to avoid predators, and hence less likely to have kin that survive.

Thus traits selected by evolution need not serve the good of the individual. Most glands an animal possesses serve the good of the individual. The pancreas enables the animal to digest food, the adrenal gland enables the animal to respond to stress, and so on. But the octopus has a self-destruct mechanism built into an optic gland. The gland has been selected because it ensures that after the mother has laid her eggs, she loses her appetite, and spends all her time guarding her brood until they can take care of themselves, at which time she dies. If this organ is surgically removed, she regains her appetite, and, ignoring her brood, may even become interested in males again. Most importantly, she may live up to nine times as long as a 'normal' female octopus after laying her eggs (Barash, 1981, p.95). Such an organ has a function, but it does not serve the mother's good.

It seems clear that there are parts of biological systems whose functions impair the good of the individuals. The optic gland of the octopus has the function of ensuring the mother concentrates on the needs of her brood at the expense of her own. The functioning of this gland does not enhance the mother's good – on the contrary, it impairs it. *Her* good is enhanced by the *interference* with the functioning of that organ (for example, by surgical excision). However, on the Evaluative Theory we would be forced to say that the optic gland has no function at all (since it does not contribute to her good), which is clearly false – it has the function of ensuring she guards her eggs.

It might be argued in reply that it only seems to us that these mechanisms do not serve the good of the individual organisms, but that this is because we are guilty of anthropomorphism. If we were octopuses, perhaps we would think that surgery would not serve our good – perhaps octopus-good consists in self-destruction in this manner. But this reply seems far-fetched. If we are to make sense of the notion of the good of an animal, it must at least have something to do with the survival of the animal, albeit its survival in a certain state – free of pain, hunger, etc.

But even if we perversely accept that octopus-good consists in its self-destruction in this manner, we would have difficulty accepting this account of our own good. For example, it is possible that ageing represents a self-destruct mechanism that has been selected by group selection. Groups composed of individuals that did not age might have rapidly outstripped the food supply, and perished. While, on the other hand, the only groups to have survived might have been those composed of individuals with the ageing self-destruct mechanism. Given this possibility, the mechanism of ageing would have a function – to ensure that the group does not grow too large and thereby outstrip the food supply.

Nevertheless, becoming more and more disabled till one finally dies is not a process that enhances the good of individual human beings. If this ageing mechanism were programmed into the pineal gland, and if the surgical removal of the pineal gland enabled us to live healthy and vigorous lives till we die of accident or disease (at the average age of 200), it would be the *disruption* of the function of the pineal gland that would serve our individual good, and not its *proper* functioning.

It might be argued that such traits and mechanisms do not have a function for the organism with them, but that they do have a function for the offspring (or group – whatever the case may be), and this *because* they serve the good of the offspring (or group). Thus the optic gland has no function for the mother, but it has a function for the offspring because it serves the good of the offspring. Similarly, it is because ageing serves the good of the group that it has a function. As long as the part contributes to the good of *some* entity, it has a function (for that entity).

But this is far too weak a criterion for attributing functions. My appendix does not have a function simply because it contributes to the good of the intestinal bacteria it houses, or because it contributes to the good of surgeons by keeping them in business! A malfunctioning car can contribute to the good of the undertakers, but this does not ensure that the defective brakes have a function!

The Evaluative Theory can make its position less trivial by requiring that biological functions serve the good of the genes. It is because the optic gland serves the good of the mother's genes (by enabling copies of them to appear in many organisms in the next generation) that it has a function. And similarly, it is because the ageing mechanism serves the good of the ageing animal's genes that it has a function.

However, there are two problems with this answer. Firstly, it is not clear that we can attribute any sense to the idea of an individual molecule having a good or well-being. It is difficult to find circumstances where we would want to say that some molecule was flourishing! And secondly, even if we can make sense of this idea, it seems a little *ad hoc* to define their good in such a way that the theory generates the right consequences. It is a fact that all biological traits with functions improve the survival chances of *copies* of the organism's genes in future generations. The Evaluative Theory could generate all the right consequences simply by defining 'the good of the genes' in terms of 'whatever increases the likelihood that another gene of the same type appeared in further generations'. But then the question arises as to why we should call this the *good* of the gene? Why should the good of a molecule be served by the existence of *other* (albeit similar) molecules in future generations? My good would certainly not be served by the existence of future clones.

Thus the Evaluative Theory is unable to provide necessary or sufficient conditions for a part to have a function. In addition, it fails to solve the philosophic puzzles that we require of our concept of function. It fails to make any distinction between effects that are mere accidents and effects that are the function of the part. On this theory, it is as much a function of my nose to support my spectacles as it is to heat and humidify the air. Similarly, it is as much a function of my heart to produce heart sounds as it is to pump blood – this is because it serves as an aid to diagnosis, and thereby serves my good.

In addition, the Evaluative Theory fails to explain how citing an effect can explain the presence of the cause. There is no benevolent law of the universe that enables us to explain the presence of a cause by its beneficial effects. The existence of my nose is explained by its heating of the air, but not by its support of spectacles. It is only if we can distinguish between accidents and functions that the attribution of a function can explain the existence of a part. The clinging potential of the Duypetrens contracture that accidentally saves my life does not explain the existence of the contracture – it is just an accident that it has this beneficial effect.

It might be argued that the Evaluative Theory can explain why the parts of some systems like the solar system do not have functions, while parts of organisms do. It is because solar systems do not have a good that can be served, while organisms do have a good, that the parts of the solar system do not have functions, while the parts of organisms do. However, this runs into problems because the parts of artefacts like cars have functions, but they do not serve the good of the individual car. Rather, they serve the good of the car's users, namely us.

But if the Evaluative Theory allows reference to some other object's good being served before we can attribute functions of the parts of certain systems, it runs into the following difficulty. If the solar system did not tend toward a state of minimal potential energy, things would not look good for us – the earth would spiral into the sun, destroying all life on earth. Thus, the achievement of this end by the solar system serves our good. But this does not mean that the parts of the solar system have a function – they do not have this effect in order to ensure that things will go well for us on earth. It seems, then, that the requirement that a system serve some good before its parts can have functions will not enable us to show why only certain systems can have parts with functions.

## The teleological theory

In this section I will examine the Teleological Theory of function. I will call any account teleological if it makes an essential reference to the property of having a goal. Such an account will have the following structure:

> The function of X (in Y) is Z if and only if (a) X does Z, and (b) X doing Z contributes to some goal of Y's.

Christopher Boorse adopts a teleological theory of function:

> 'X is performing the function Z in the G-ing of S at t' *means* 'At t, X is Z-ing and the Z-ing of X is making a causal contribution to the goal G or the goal-directed system S' (Boorse, 1976a, p.80)

But the Teleological Theory also cannot provide necessary and sufficient conditions for having a function. It cannot provide sufficient conditions for having a function because there are effects of parts that accidentally contribute to the goals of their systems, but which are not thereby the functions of those parts. Flat feet might enable me to serve my goal of survival by avoiding the army, but it is not the function of my flat feet to enable me to survive. Andrew Woodfield tells the following story:

> Suppose that the dog's stomach rumbled, thereby helping the dog to achieve some goal it happened to have, like frightening away a cat. Rumbling would not count as a function of the stomach on the strength of that (Woodfield, 1976, p.126).

The theory does not seem to provide necessary conditions either. There are objects that have functions but which nevertheless do not contribute to any goals. Artefacts such as chairs have functions but are not part of goal-directed systems. As Larry Wright argues:

> On the other hand, many things have *functions* (for example chairs and windpipes) which do not behave *at all*, much less goal-directedly. And behaviour can have a function without being goal directed – for example, pacing the floor or blinking your eye (Wright, 1973, p.140).

Here it seems fair to reply that it is the system of the artefacts plus their makers (us) that is goal-directed. For example, chairs contribute to the goal of seating humans. As Christopher Boorse argues:

> Artefacts, by contrast, may or may not be goal-directed in and of themselves. Thermostats and guided missiles are; chairs and fountain pens are not. But we do attribute functions to chairs and fountain pens and to their parts, and I think we do so by taking the artefact together with its purposive human user as a goal-directed system. Pens have functions because they contribute to the goal-directed human activity of writing. Such objects, which lack the appropriate organization to be independent centres of teleology, must inherit their functional features from people's use of them (Boorse, 1976a, 80).

While the Teleological Theory avoids this problem, it generates others. If chairs can have a function because they serve our goal of sitting, how do we avoid the conclusion that the ozone layer of the atmosphere has a function because it serves our goal of survival by protecting us from dangerous ultraviolet light? The more ultraviolet light from which we need protection, the more the ozone layer is formed, thereby achieving the goal of enabling us to survive. But the ozone layer does not have a function – it is a happy accident that it contributes to our goal of survival. So the Teleological Theory cannot solve the problem of artifactual functions in this way without generating other difficulties.

The Teleological Theory runs into difficulty because there are problems with giving an account of what it is to be a goal of a system. The goals of systems are standardly specified in terms of the end state to which the system is directed. Our lives seem to be directed towards our survival into old age. But what is there to prevent us from saying that the goal of life is to *die* of old age? The systems of our bodies would then all be serving this goal. But would it be correct to say that their function is to enable us to die of old age?

Even if this problem could be solved, and we could show that this is not the goal of (human) life, functions do not have anything to do with goals. Fresh-water plankton diurnally vary their distance below the surface of the water. This behaviour is directed towards the end-state of keeping the intensity of light constant. But it is not the function of the behaviour to keep the light intensity constant. The function is to keep the oxygen supply (which happens to vary with the intensity of sunlight) constant (Wright, 1973, p.140).

The theory is also not able to solve the philosophic puzzles with which we began. It is not able to draw the distinction between accidents and functions – it is as much the function (on this theory) of the heart to produce heart sounds (they contribute to survival by enabling physicians to better diagnose illness) as it is to pump blood. It is as much the function of my nose to support glasses as it is to heat and humidify the air.

Nor can the Teleological Theory explain why it is that citing the function of an item can explain its presence. Since there is no teleological law that ensures that if something will contribute to some goal, it will exist, the existence of an item is not explained by citing its function (on this account of function).

In order for the Teleological Theory to solve Nagel's problem, it has to give an account to what it is to be a goal-directed system such that we can show that solar systems are not goal-directed, while organisms are. Even if it can, it will not avoid the basic difficulty that functions do not seem to have anything to do with goals.

### The aetiological theory

In this section we will see whether the Aetiological Theory can give an account of our concept of function. Such an account will have the following structure:

The function of X (in Y) is Z if and only if (a) X does Z, and (b) X doing Z makes a causal contribution to X's occurrence in Y.

Larry Wright proposes an Aetiological Theory:

> The function of X is Z *means* (a) X is there because it does Z, (b) Z is a consequence (result) of X's being there (Wright, 1973, p.161).

Similarly, Jonathan Bennett advocates an aetiological view:

> 'The function of the mammalian heart is to pump blood throughout the body' means (a) The mammalian heart does pump blood throughout the body, and (b) The fact that mammals have hearts is explained by the fact that hearts pump blood throughout the body (a mutant which lacked a heart would not survive because its blood would not circulate) (Bennett, 1976, p.79).

When we say that hearts have the function of pumping blood, we are saying nothing other than that hearts pump blood and that that is the reason why we have them. Similarly, to say that the function of spark plugs is to ignite fuel is to say that spark plugs do this and that this is the reason why spark plugs have been included in cars. It is clear that we require no reference to the good of the system or the goal of the system. All that is needed is that certain causal connections occur.

We can now see why the Duypetrens contracture that saves my life does not have a function – it is not included in my body because of the effect that it has. Similarly, the loose nut does not have the function of adjusting the valve because the loose nut is not there because it has this effect – it is there just by accident. In this way the Aetiological Theory can draw a distinction between accidents and functions. It is not the function of the nose to support spectacles because this effect does not play a causal role in the explanation of why we have noses. On the other hand, it is the function of the nose to heat and humidify the air because this effect *did* have a causal role in our coming to have noses.

The Aetiological Theory is also able to show why having a certain function can explain the presence of that item. It follows by definition (on this view) that if an item has a function, then this was instrumental (in some way) in that item coming to exist in the system. The theory is also able to explain why parts of the solar system do not have functions. It is only systems with parts whose effects have a causal role in explaining the presence of those parts in

109

the systems that can have functions. The parts of the solar system (and the behaviour of the solar system) are not there (do not occur) because of some effect they have. And because of this, the parts do not have functions. Of course, if God had included a planet because of some effect it had on the solar system, the planet *would* have a part with a function. But this is only because it now satisfies the aetiological schema.

Finally, the theory shows that hearts have a function in the same sense that spark-plugs have a function. The heart has a function of pumping blood because it does so and its doing so plays a causal role in explaining (via natural selection) why mammals have hearts. And spark-plugs have the function of igniting fuel because they do so and their doing so plays a causal role (via the intention of the agents who designed and built the car) in explaining why cars have them. In both cases the truth conditions of attributing functions consist in certain causal connections.

I want now to discuss and rebut certain proposed counter-examples to the Aetiological Theory. The first is the problem of the *first mutant*. The very first organism with a heart would not have had the heart because of its ability to pump blood, but because of the chance mutation of its genes. So on the Aetiological Theory the first heart would not have had a function. But it may be felt that it has no less a function when it first appears than after it has been selected.

We cannot avoid this problem by arguing that as soon as the mutant heart exerts a causal effect on the survival of the individual, its presence in him at a later time *is* in part explained by the ability of the heart to pump blood at an earlier time – if it did not have the ability, the first mutant would have died. But this will not work for traits like the peacock's plumage – this is because such traits do *not* explain how it is that the same organism survives to possess that trait – on the contrary, those with the trait are less likely to survive (because it attracts predators).

But the first mutant's organ only *seems* to have a function because we let our knowledge of what happens afterwards to bias our judgment. Were we to encounter a trait that has some beneficial effect in a mutant, but is never selected, we are not tempted to think that the effect was the function of the trait. If we encountered an animal with the trait of a noisy stomach, we would not think this had a function, even if it scared off a predator. But we might be tempted to think that this first noisy stomach did have a function if we knew that this trait was later to be incorporated into members of that species by natural selection.

The question then arises at what stage the Aetiological Theory is prepared to say that the organ has a function. I think the organ acquires a function when its appearance *in the next generation* is (in part) the result of some effect of that organ. The organ or trait in question does not have to spread throughout the species by natural selection before it acquires a function. Sickle-cell trait is possessed by those who have a single gene that codes for the abnormal haemoglobin molecule. The red cells of such individuals enable them to resist malarial parasitization, and have been selected for this reason in populations living in malarial areas. However, the trait is unlikely ever to be possessed by all members of any population, because individuals with a double dose of the gene suffer from sickle-cell anaemia. Nevertheless, sickle-cell trait has a function.

The second problem is that of the *crazy breeder*. Suppose a hereditary condition C of mice causes them to be in constant pain. A crazy breeder might kill all those who do not have this condition, thereby artificially selecting those with C. On the Aetiological Theory we are forced to say that C has the function of producing pain – because all those who are not in pain are killed by the crazy breeder. But this might sound unattractive to those who think that such a condition cannot have a function.

But C does have a function – we only *think* that it does not because we mistakenly believe that all functions must serve the good of the individual organism – and we have seen that this is not so. It is often difficult to accept some functional ascription until we know how the trait came to be selected – until we know the special circumstances in which the trait conferred an evolutionary advantage. For example, it is difficult to accept that the function of the male praying mantis's sexual overtures is to get his head chopped off by his mate. But when we learn that he can only copulate effectively when he has 'lost his head' – the cerebral ganglion, perhaps like the inhibitory cerebral cortex in man, exerts an inhibitory effect on the abdominal ganglion controlling copulation, and this arrangement has been selected so that he provides his future offspring with a solid meal, we can accept the functional ascription (Manning, 1979, p.14).

The third problem is that of the *systems without histories*. As Christopher Boorse argues:

Suppose we discovered, for example, that at some point the lion species simply sprang into existence by an unparalleled saltation [global mutation]. One would not regard this discovery as invalidating all function claims about lions; it would show that in at least one case an intricate functional organisation was created by chance. Given a little knowledge about what happens inside mammals, it is obvious that the function of the heart is to circulate blood. That is what the heart contributes to the organism's overall goals, rather than its weight or noise. But it cannot be obvious in any strict sense that the heart had an aetiology in which this effect rather than the others played a role. Nothing about the aetiology of the heart is obvious on inspection at all (Boorse, 1976a, p.75).

A variant of this argument is Richard Sorabji's case of *luxury functions:*

Suppose that an organ were discovered which came into operation only when some lethal type of damage had occurred, eg., a major coronary thrombosis. And suppose that the effect of this organ were to shut off sensations of pain as soon as such lethal damage had occurred. This effect would not increase the chances of survival either for individual or for species. But it would confer a good of another sort. For the shutting off of unnecessary pain is a good. And it would be perfectly correct to say that the function of the organ was to shut off pain when lethal damage had occurred (Sorabji, 1964, p.293).

In both examples, it is argued that the organs have functions in the absence of the relevant aetiology for those organs.

But organs cannot have functions without the relevant aetiology – we can only discover what these functions are when we discover the aetiology. This becomes clear if we consider unfamiliar systems where we will not be influenced by our background knowledge. Suppose strange machines that dismantle themselves begin materializing on earth. How do we decide what functions the parts serve? Do the parts have the function of contributing to the goal of dismantling the machine, puzzling us, providing us with spare parts, increasing the entropy of the universe, messing up the earth, or something else? Since there is no way we can decide among these alternatives, we cannot say what the function of the machines (or their parts) are. And this is precisely because we do not have access to their aetiology. If we knew that they were designed by extraterrestrials to amuse us, then we would be able to ascribe functions to them, but this only because we know the reason why the parts had been included. Knowing the aetiology is *essential* for correctly ascribing functions.

In addition, when biologists look for the function of a trait, they look for the aetiology for that trait. For example, discovering the function of 'alarm calls' entails looking for the explanation why such a trait came to be selected. For the alarm call has many effects – warning the group, drawing attention of the predator to the caller, manipulating the group to flee the predator, and so on – but to discover its function is to discover which of those effects was instrumental in getting such a trait selected.

Paul Sherman argues that alarm calls in Belding's ground squirrels have the function of warning kin. If, as I have argued, this implies that the trait of giving warning calls evolved in a certain way, we should find Sherman arguing that it is because the trait has evolved via kin selection that it has such a function. He writes:

> My investigation indicates that assisting relatives, nepotism, is the most likely function of the ground squirrels' alarm call; this result implicates kin selection in the evolution of a behaviour that, because it may involve risks to the alarm caller's phenotype, appears to be altruistic (Sherman, 1977, p.1249).

Two biologists, Charnov and Krebs, in an article 'Evolution of alarm calls: altruism or manipulation?', argue that alarm calls have the function of manipulating the group because this was how the trait came to be selected:

> We propose that the calling habit spread because of a positive benefit associated with calling. The individual seeing the hawk would seem to be in a good position to avoid being caught by *manipulating* its flock mates. Having seen the hawk, the bird has two pieces of information: that there is a hawk, and the position of the hawk. If the caller passes on only part of this information to its flock mates, it will be able to use them to enhance its own safety. The non-callers are simply told that there is a hawk, and head for cover without regard to the predator's direction of approach. The caller can now protect

itself by 'seeking cover' on the far side or the middle of the flock (Charnov and Krebs, 1975, p.110).

Again, the argument is that the trait has such a function because it was through this effect that it got there.

Nicholas Smythe argues that the function of alarm calls is to induce the predators to attack because (again) this was the reason why they were selected:

> I do not question that such signals may often carry information that is of use to conspecifics. However, I believe that their evolution occurred in a different context, that, under certain circumstances, potential prey animals may actually gain an advantage from advertising their whereabouts to potential predators as conspicuously as possible, with the object of inducing the predators to [prematurely] attack (Smythe, 1970, p.491).

Thus biologists look for the *aetiology* of the trait when they try to discover its function. So I would argue that Boorse is simply wrong to assume that we do not need facts about aetiology before we can ascribe functions correctly. And Sorabji is also wrong – if the luxury organ has no relevant aetiology, then it simply has no function.

The next problem is that of the *lost function*. Suppose the appendix came to be selected because it housed bacteria that were needed to digest grass. However, in humans, since we don't eat grass, the appendix has no function, or it has lost its function. But on the Aetiological Theory we have to say that it (still) has a function, because its effect played a causal role in its coming to be in mammals. To avoid these cases, we must amend the account of function as follows:

> The function of X (in Y) is Z if and only if (a) X does Z, and (b) X doing Y makes a causal contribution to X's *continued presence* in Y.

With this modification, the problem can be avoided – it is because hearts continue to exert their causal role in being maintained in vertebrates that hearts still have a function. On the other hand, it is because appendices do not continue to exert a causal role in being retained in humans that they have lost their function.

This move also solves the problem of *altered functions*. The lungs of reptiles probably developed from swim bladders of fish. There must then have been a time when one and the same organ changed its function. Although the organ came to be there because of one of its effects (namely, to enable fish to alter their water level), it continued to be there because of a different one (namely, to enable fish to breathe air).

The aetiological account faces two more difficult problems. Firstly, the problem of *inorganic evolution*. Suppose at the beginning of the earth's history there are a number of different mountains, some made of granite, some of sandstone, some with forests covering them, some without, and so on. Over the years, the forces of nature ensure that some are worn away and others remain. On the Aetiological Theory, we will have to say that the function of being made of granite is to resist erosion – granite resists erosion, and it's this that explains why the mountain remains and continues to have the property of being made of granite.

The second problem is that of the *deviant causal chain*. Christopher Boorse raised the problem:

> A hornet buzzing in a woodshed so frightens a farmer that he
> repeatedly shrinks from going in and killing it. Nothing in
> Wright's essay blocks the conclusion that the function of the
> buzzing, or even of the hornet, is to frighten the farmer. The
> farmer's fright is a result of the hornet's presence, and the
> hornet's presence continues because it has this result. ...
> Obesity in a man of meagre motivation can prevent him from
> exercising. Although failure to exercise is a result of the
> obesity, and the obesity continues because of this result, it is
> unlikely that prevention of exercise is its function (Boorse,
> 1976a, p.75).

Many neurotic defence mechanisms are self-maintaining – defence against anxiety is often productive of more anxiety, which explains why the neurotic defences persist. But the function of the defence mechanism is not to produce anxiety. Again, if a society began to burn books, and tnis results in ignorance which perpetuated the ritual of book-burning, it would be wrong to say that the ritual had the function of producing ignorance.

It might be thought that we can avoid these problems if we

require the causal chain to proceed via the enhancement of some entity's good before the part can have a function. But this is wrong. Psychiatrists might encourage the persistence of neuroses in their patients because this enables them to make a lot of money – neuroses enhance the good of the psychiatrists, and they continue to be there (in neurotics) because they have this effect. But it is not their function to make money for psychiatrists.

Just as we can have vicious causal circles, we can have virtuous causal circles – a person's happiness can lead to his making many friends – everybody likes people who are cheerful, and few like those who are always depressed. And a person's having many friends might further contribute to his happiness. But it would be wrong to conclude that the function of happiness is to enable one to make friends.

The best solution to these problems is to exclude causal chains of the wrong sort. I suggest we amend the theory as follows:

> The function of X (in Y) is Z if and only if (a) X does Z and (b) X doing Z makes a causal contribution to X's continued presence in Y *in the right sort of way.*

This account has the virtues of excluding such counter examples – the parts in question are not there because of causal chains of the right sort, like biological parts that are there via natural selection, or parts of artefacts that are there via the intentions of agents. It also shows what is common among functions that arise naturally (natural functions) and those that arise via the intentions of agents (intentional functions).

The account does not assume that knowing the exact mechanism is part of knowing the meaning of the term – it is up to biologists to discover the details. Like our concept of perception, where we do not take someone to have perceived an object unless he is in the right sort of causal relation with this object, we are not required to know the details of what this right sort of causal relation consists in in order to possess the concept – we just need to know that there is some mechanism that underlies genuine perception. We certainly do not want to say that those who believed that organisms were designed by God did not have the concept of function – as long as they believed that there was *some* mechanism of the right sort, we must take them to have possessed the concept, even though they were wrong about the mechanism. As Jonathan Bennett remarks:

Where the functional statement concerns an organism, I believe that the explanation will always be an evolutionary one, but that it is no part of the meaning of the functional statement. Someone who says 'The function of the grass's movement is to get sunlight' might think that the relevant explanation is theological: God implanted the requisite mechanism in grass because he wanted it to get sunlight. Or he might have some other sort of explanation in mind; or indeed, he may have no opinion about the explanation except that there is one (Bennett, 1976, p.79).

What I want to do now is to develop the account of what these mechanisms consist in. Let us start with what I have called intentional functions. In the case of artefacts, the 'right sort of way' might be unpacked like this:

The function of X (in Y) is Z if and only if (a) X does Z, and (b) X doing Z makes a causal contribution to X's continued presence in Y via some agent's intention of include X in Y for that purpose.

This account explains why spark-plugs have a function – they ignite fuel and agents include them in cars because they have this effect. It also explains the following example.

Suppose an agent intends to blow up a building, but fails to connect the bomb correctly. However, his aims make him nervous, he perspires into the bomb leaving a saline solution that enables the detonator to set off the bomb. We would not say that the function of this perspiration was to conduct the detonating charge even though it did so, and the presence of the perspiration in the bomb was the result of the agent's intention to blow up the building. And this because it was not included in the right sort of way.

Let us turn to the task of developing the account of natural functions (functions not acquired through the intentions of agents). We might expand 'the right sort of way' like this:

The function of X (in Y) is Z if and only if (a) X does Z, and (b) X doing Z makes a causal contribution to X's continued presence in Y via the mechanism of natural selection.

This shows that all the putative counterexamples fail because they are not cases underpinned by natural selection. The case of obesity, acquiring friends, the neurotic defence, the buzzing hornet, the surviving mountains, and the ritual of burning books do not have functions because the causal chain did not proceed via the mechanism of natural selection.

This account does not exclude entities besides organisms from acquiring functions without the intentions of agents. For example, if machines could make copies of themselves, they could evolve and come to have parts with natural functions. This is an interesting consequence of the theory, and one I think we should accept. Neither does the account exclude features of social organization from having natural functions. If we define 'natural selection' more abstractly, we can think of rituals and so on as acquiring natural functions. For example, a ritual might have the (natural) function of ensuring social cohesion. This is because it has this effect, and because it continues to be in societies because of this effect. This may have arisen because those societies without the ritual did not survive and spread, so that the surviving societies came to have the ritual.

If we adopt a liberal reading of 'natural selection', we can explain why it is we might be tempted to think of such features as having (natural) functions. Given that natural selection (among organisms) occurs because they are able to reproduce themselves (natural selection occurs by definition when one sort of organism leaves more offspring than another), extensions of the concept will be most plausible when we have entitites that are able to 'reproduce' themselves in some way. For example, machines and societies in the examples above. However, in the problem of inorganic evolution, we are not tempted to think of the parts of mountains as having functions because here we do not have natural selection at work – mountains do not reproduce themselves.

Thus I think that the best account that we can provide of the concept of function is one provided by the Aetiological Theory. It is able to provide necessary and sufficient conditions for having a function. In addition, it is able to solve the philosophic problems facing any account of function. It is also able to explain why we are prepared to extend the concept of natural functions in certain directions and not in others.

Most importantly for our purposes, we can see that the account of function is value-free – no essential reference to the good of the system is required before we can attribute a function. A part can have a function in a system without its serving the good of that system. On the contrary, we have seen that the functions of many parts impair the good of the system in which they occur. In addition, the account of function is objective – no reference is needed to subjective factors such as personal values, preferences, or decisions before we can attribute any function. There is an objective and value-free fact of the matter whether a part has a function, and just what that function is – we can discover this by investigating the aetiology of the system. Our next task is to see whether the concept of function, or rather, malfunction, can elucidate the concept of disease.

# CHAPTER 7
# THE NATURALIST THEORY

## Introduction

Thomas Szasz argues that the concept of disease implies a deviation from some clearly defined norm. He feels that the norm for physical illness is objective, but questions the objectivity of the norm for mental illnesses:

> In the case of physical illness, the norm is the structural and functional integrity of the human body. Thus although the desirability of physical health, as such, is an ethical value, what health is can be stated in anatomical and physiological terms. What is the norm deviation from which is regarded as mental illness (Szasz, 1960, p.114)?

There appears to be a problem in the domain of mental illness because it seems more open to subjectivism: norms of healthy conduct can be selected at will to turn any undesirable or non-conformist behaviour into a mental illness. Take one psychiatrist's account of mental health: 'Mental health consists in the ability to live happily, productively, without being a nuisance' (Wootton, 1959, p.98)! Any non-conformist could legitimately be labelled as mentally ill on such an account of normality.

Aubrey Lewis, the great British psychiatrist, perceiving this difficulty, argued that such non-conformist behaviour was only pathological if it was due to the disturbance of the function of some psychological part. For mental illness to be inferred:

> disorder of function must be detectable at a discrete or differentiated level that is hardly conceivable when mental activity as a whole is taken as the irreducible datum. If non-conformity can be detected only in total behaviour, while all

the particular psychological functions seem unimpaired, health will be presumed not illness (Lewis, 1955, p.118).

Thus an attractive solution to the problem of subjectivism in psychiatric classification is offered by the account of the concept of disease in terms of the disruption of function. It is only when the behaviour is due to the disruption of some psychological function that it is due to some disease. Only if non-conformity is due to some malfunction will the person be diseased. We can thereby avoid the subjectivity of using such accounts of norms in terms of 'being a nuisance'. Since it will be an objective fact of the matter as to what are the functions of the brain (rather than a subjective matter as to what is a nuisance), it will be an objective fact of the matter as to what are disruptions of part-functions (and hence diseases).

The account of disease in terms of malfunction is attractive, but is it right? This is the issue I will examine in this chapter. This will complete the evalution of the Naturalist thesis that the concept of disease is to be understood in terms of the value-free concept of malfunction.

On the face of it, the account of disease in terms of the disruption of function seems plausible. It is easy to make the mistake of thinking that deciduous trees are diseased if one does not know they are deciduous – the yellowing of leaves mimics a disease. It is the discovery that the loss of leaves has a function that enables one to conclude that the trees are not ill. When we see a gall-midge being eaten alive from the inside by smaller organisms, we tend to think that the gall-midge must be suffering from some disease. However, when we then learn that the mother lays her eggs inside herself to provide her offspring with their first meal (that is, it has a function), we realize she is not suffering from any disease. It is the discovery that there is no malfunction that enables one to conclude that she is not ill.

The plan of the chapter is as follows: I will firstly give an account of the notion of malfunction, and then go on to give an account of the concept of disease (and pathology) in terms of this concept. Finally, I will assess whether this account can withstand certain objections.

## The concept of malfunction

In Chapter 6 I argued for the following account of the concept of function:

121

The function of X (in Y) is Z if and only if (a) X does Z, and (b) X doing Z makes a causal contribution to X's continued presence in Y in the right sort of way.

We also provided expansions of this account for both intentional functions and natural (biological) functions. For the latter, the 'right sort of way' was interpreted as 'via the mechanism of natural selection'.

Not all biological systems with functions need have been selected by evolution. A biological system can have either a natural or an intentional function. For example, the function of the mammalian heart is a natural function because the heart is in the mammal via the mechanism of natural selection.

On the other hand, suppose a gene coding for infra-red photoreceptors was introduced by genetic engineers into our genome, such that it enabled us to see in the dark. These photoreceptors would have a function, but it would be an intentional one – the photoreceptors are not there via the mechanism of natural selection. They are there via the intention of the genetic engineers. So the parts of biological systems can have intentional functions as well as natural ones.

Just as parts that have natural functions need not necessarily serve the good of the individual organism, so genetically engineered parts with intentional functions need not serve the good of the individual. A mad dictator might get his genetic engineers to programme his subjects with an auto-destruct system which operated when they ceased to be economically useful. Such a system would have a function, but it would not serve the good of the individual.

In order to judge whether some organism has a malfunction, we have to judge his functional capacity in relation to the appropriate reference group. If bats fail to locate objects with sound, they are malfunctioning. But are we malfunctioning when we are not able to locate objects in this way? Are we malfunctioning because we cannot fly? Obviously not. This means that an animal does not have a malfunction if it simply lacks some functional ability. An organism only has a malfunction if its functional capacity falls below that of members of the same species.

Of course this will not do as it stands. This is because different sexes and different stages of the same species do not have the same functional abilities. A caterpillar is not malfunctioning simply because it cannot fly, and a man is not malfunctioning simply because be cannot breast feed. So an organism only has a malfunction if its functional capacity falls below that of members of the same species at the same stage and of the same sex.

However, this will not do either. Pygmy women have a unique method of storing energy – they have the capacity to store fat in their buttocks, producing large protuberant fat stores known as steatopygia. These have the function of enabling them to survive for long periods without food, but they are not systems that are characteristic of all females of the human species. However, the trait is characteristic of the race of pygmies. A pygmy woman unable to store food in this way will be malfunctioning. On the other hand, my wife (thank goodness) is not malfunctioning simply because she is unable to store food in this way!

Similarly, aborigines have acquired various adaptations that enable them to survive in areas with little water. Their stomachs have the ability to act as water bottles, storing large quantities of water. An aborigine failing to store water in this way would be malfunctioning, but other humans are not malfunctioning because they lack this ability. An organism only has a malfunction if its functional ability falls below other members of the same race at the same stage and of the same sex.

However, not all members of a particular race will have the same functional abilities. There is a Saharan tribe whose members possess kidneys that are better able to concentrate urine (and thereby conserve water loss) than other members of the same race. But other members of their race are not thereby malfunctioning. An organism only has a malfunction if its functional ability falls below other members of the same interbreeding population at the same stage and of the same sex.

However, we can imagine someone with sickle-cell trait (living in a malarial-infested region) acquiring a viral infection that interferes with the functioning of this trait, such that his red blood cells are no longer able to resist malarial parasitization. He has a malfunction even though we know that not all members of his interbreeding population can acquire sickle-cell trait (the double dose of the gene is lethal because it leads to sickle-cell anaemia).

We cannot define a malfunction relative to a subgroup of an interbreeding population. This would mean that we could not say that albinos, for example, had a malfunction because relative to some subgroup of the interbreeding population (namely, those consisting of albinos), they do not lack any functional ability! In order to avoid this difficulty, we must distinguish two types of malfunction.

There are two kinds of malfunctions organisms can have. One is an acquired malfunction, and the other is a hereditary one. An organism has an acquired malfunction if and only if it has acquired a system with a function, and some environmental factor interferes with its production of this function. This entails that the individual with the viral infection interfering with the anti-malarial action of his sickle cells has an acquired malfunction.

An organism has a hereditary malfunction if and only if it has a hereditary lack of a system with a function possessed by the vast majority of members of its interbreeding population at the same stage and of the same sex. This entails that humans who are colour blind have a hereditary malfunction, and albinos who lack the ability to synthesize melanin have a hereditary malfunction. It also explains why we do not take those who lack sickle-cell trait to have a hereditary malfunction – the vast majority of members of any interbreeding population do not have the trait, and therefore its lack does not count as a hereditary malfunction.

This account of biological malfunctions shows us that what is and is not a malfunction is relative to the population in which the individual exists. For example, if a pygmy were to develop a sensitivity to growth hormone, we would say that he had developed some malfunction. This is because all pygmies have an insensitivity to growth hormone which (I assume) has a function, perhaps of enabling them to remain concealed from prey in the shrubs. While a Masai's sensitivity to growth hormone does not amount to his having a malfunction! This is because in him it is the sensitivity to growth hormone that has a function – of enabling him to keep tall and cool.

On this account it is possible for all members of a species (or subspecies) to have a particular malfunction. This is easily seen with acquired malfunctions. We can imagine all of us succumbing to AIDS. In addition, we can imagine ourselves discovering that we are *now* all suffering from some malfunction. We may discover that we all have minute traces of lead in our bodies which we inhale from automobile fumes. We may discover that these minute traces of lead impair our hearing and sight – when they are removed, our visual and auditory acuity is greatly enhanced. Thus we might come to have evidence that we are all presently malfunctioning.

It is also possible to imagine a whole species coming to have a particular hereditary malfunction. Humans have lost the ability to synthesize vitamin C – this is a trait possessed by the animals from which we have evolved. Suppose this happened as a result of a Velikovsky-like catastrophe which killed all our ancestors who had this ability, but left alive those few defective ones who lacked it. If we took the reference group to include the dead organisms as well, we can conclude that all the surviving members of the species would have a hereditary malfunction.

Not all departures from the typical functional capacity will count as a malfunction. Suppose that the function of the heart is to pump 5 litres of blood per minute – it is this ability that explains why it is there. But if a heart pumps 7 litres of blood per minute, it will hardly be malfunctioning! It is because the heart has been selected for its capacity to pump at such an output *or more* that its pumping more does not count as a malfunction – on the contrary, this counts as the heart's hyperfunctioning.

Not all interferences with the functioning of some biological system will produce malfunctions – the interference in the functioning might itself have a function. We have a system that secretes endogenous opiates called 'endorphines' that interferes with the perception of pain and thereby enables us to ignore pain in emergencies. This system might be thought of as producing a malfunction of our pain perceiving apparatus. But even though the function of the pain perceiving apparatus is to perceive pain, it is no less its function to be sensitive to being damped by endorphines – a pain perceiving mechanism *failing* to be damped would be malfunctioning. So where the sensitivity to interference has itself been selected, it would be wrong to see the interference as producing a malfunction.

In summary, I have argued that there are two sorts of malfunctions. While one can have an acquired malfunction of a part that is not possessed by all members of the population (or species), it is not possible to have a hereditary malfunction of a part that is not population- or species-typical. It is now time to turn to the account of diseases in terms of this concept.

## Disease as malfunctioning

I have already argued that we cannot give necessary and sufficient conditions for the concept of disease – it is a family resemblance one. The thesis I wish to examine now is that being a process productive of a malfunction is a necessary condition for being a disease, and a sufficient condition for being pathological. I will argue that both these theses are mistaken.

There is at least one necessary condition for being a disease, and this is the property of being a process. In contexts where the explanation for a condition is not obvious, we are likely to classify the underlying process as a disease. This would lead us to expect that in *such contexts*, being a process productive of a malfunction would be necessary *and* sufficient for being a disease. This too is wrong.

Christopher Boorse is the main exponent of this theory of disease. He puts his position thus:

> An organism is *healthy* at any moment in proportion as it is not diseased; and a *disease* is a type of internal state of the organism which (i) interferes with the performance of some natural function – i.e. some species-typical contribution to survival and reproduction – characteristic of the organism's age; and (ii) is not simply in the nature of the species, i.e., is either atypical of the species or, if typical, mainly due to environmental causes (Boorse, 1976b, p.62).

He goes on to emphasize that this definition makes a number of points:

> First, diseases are interferences with natural functions. Second, since the functional organization typical of a species is a biological fact, the concept of disease is value-free. Whether or not an organism is diseased can be settled in principle by the methods of natural science (Boorse, 1976b, p.62).

Boorse is correct to point out that on such an account of the concept of disease, there is a value-free fact of the matter whether an organism is malfunctioning (that is, diseased). This means that we will be able to avoid the spectre of subjectivism. We noticed this problem especially in relation to classifying mental illnesses – unless we could provide an objective account, anyone was free to classify undesirable or non-conformist behaviour as some mental illness. But if we have an account of disease, like Lewis and Boorse offer, in terms of the notion of malfunction, we will be able to avoid this problem.

126

This account of disease has a number of virtues. Firstly, it can explain why it is that standard cases of disease – TB, multiple sclerosis, muscular dystrophy, leprosy, etc., are classified as diseases. They are all processes that produce malfunctioning. And it can explain why standard cases of other pathological conditions – myopia, club foot, carbon-monoxide poisoning, etc., are so classified – they are all conditions that produce malfunctioning.

Secondly, it explains why those who just have a statistically low functional capacity are considered to be diseased. For example, someone with a thyroid gland that produces less thyroxin than normal still has a disease (myxoedema) even though he just falls at one end of the normal distribution.

Thirdly, it explains why we refer to certain biological facts in order to decide whether some organism has a disease or not. For example, the wasting of the mother octopus, the infestation of the mother gall-midge, the infestation of the mimosa tree, all look like disease processes at work until we discover that there is no malfunctioning present. What determines whether a condition is pathological is the existence of a malfunction, and this is exactly what this account of disease predicts.

Fourthly, the account can explain how there can be diseases without symptoms. A person can have a benign lipoma, and not have any complaints. In addition, a person with early lung cancer has a disease even though he may be asymptomatic.

Fifthly, this account explains how plants and animals can have diseases, and why we refer to biological facts to make such judgments. Whether a plant is diseased or not seems to depend on whether it has a malfunction, and not on anything else.

Sixthly, the account can show that there is a difference between a condition that is a disease, and a condition it is desirable to be without. It might be desirable to be without a need for sleep, but this is not a disease. It might be desirable to be without the enzyme system for synthesizing uric acid, for this makes us liable to suffer from gout. But it is not a disease or pathological state to have such an enzyme system. It is only where a condition produces an impairment of species-typical functioning, as for example with haemophilia, that the undesirable condition is a disease.

Finally, the account enables us to avoid the problem of Relativism. Whether something is a disease does not depend on what values one affirms – it depends instead on biological facts. Of course, whether a condition is a disease will depend on what species (or population) the individual with the condition belongs to. But all this demonstrates is the *relational* character of the notion of disease. Relativism, on the other hand, is the thesis that different cultures can disagree about whether a condition is a disease, and both be correct. But on this theory, such a problem is avoided – whether some condition is a disease or not depends on certain biological facts which different cultures can agree upon. All we have to discover is whether some system has a function, and whether this is being interfered with, and there is nothing further we need to do to enable us to decide whether the condition is a disease.

In addition, this Naturalist Theory can explain why different cultural values lead to differences in disease classification. The running away of slaves, for example, is classified as the disease drapetomania, not because the concept of disease is an evaluative one, and because such behaviour was found undesirable. Rather, the concept of disease is value-free, but cultural values lead people to *believe* that certain conditions are the product of malfunctioning. It is cosy to believe that things that one does not approve of are due to malfunctioning, and all the things that one does approve of represent the body's proper functioning.

In spite of all these virtues, this account of disease and of pathological conditions is mistaken.

## Objections

It may be objected that this account is mistaken because Western civilization has possessed the concept of disease for thousands of years, but has not possessed such a sophisticated concept of function. But they have certainly been talking about diseases.

But this objection fails because one does not need to know about the mechanism of natural selection before one can possess the concept of function. Just as someone can possess the concept of perception without knowing the details of the neurophysiological mechanism of perception, so one can possess the concept of function without knowing the details of the mechanism of natural selection. To have the concept of function one need only know that parts with functions come to be in the system in the right sort of way. In the days before evolutionary theory, this mechanism was thought to be divine design.

It may be objected that an individual might have a process which in him luckily does not produce a malfunction. The individual would still have a disease, but *ex hypothesi* he does not have a malfunction. For example, he might have a benign tumour that grows slowly enough and in a safe enough site that it does not cause any malfunction. Here we feel that the individual still has a disease even though there is no malfunction. But we can avoid this objection if we define disease in terms of a process *of a type* that (in standard circumstances) results in a malfunction. The person with the benign tumour has a disease because the process is of a type that usually results in some malfunction.

The Naturalist account is mistaken for the following reasons. It cannot provide a necessary condition for being pathological or for being a disease. Suppose that natural selection endows us with an organ that secretes destructive enzymes into our bodies and leads to a painful death. The organ is there in order to ensure that the population size does not outstrip the resources – the organ comes into operation when the population reaches a certain size. The process, then, has a function (of regulating population size), but we would nevertheless not regard such a process as a disease. Being productive of malfunction is not a necessary condition for being a disease.

William Goosens also makes this point:

> Suppose in an intelligent and reflective species a structure evolved which, about twenty years after sexual maturity, altered the immunological system so that blood cells destructively attacked the membrane of the brain. The individuals, let us suppose, suffer greatly and eventually die. Surely they die of a hideous genetic disease, whose only distinction from others is its timing, latency, and frequency. It makes no difference to this judgment if we add that the condition was spread by natural selection and that it continues to promote the reproduction of the individual and even the survival of the species (Goosens, 1980, p.112).

Jonathan Barnes points out that such an objection is flawed (Jonathan Barnes in conversation). It might be conceded that a self-destruct system might have the function of keeping the population down. But it might be argued that such a system might function by causing a malfunction in some other system. It does not follow from the fact that some self-destruct system has a function that it does not cause any malfunction. If the self-destruct mechanism operates by interfering with the contraction of the heart, what is to stop us from saying that it functions by causing a cardiac *malfunction?* And if this is so, then we can conclude that the condition is a disease because there *is* a malfunction present.

But this move will not be open to us in all cases. The heart might have a *dual* function. One function is to pump blood, and the other is to be susceptible to being stopped by the self-destruct mechanism. Hearts can have this latter function because those hearts that were not susceptible were selected against. So the organism will *not* be malfunctioning when it self-destructs. We cannot then say that the self-destruct organ causes the heart to malfunction – part of the function of the heart is to stop pumping when the self-destruct organ begins operating. Much like the pain-perceiving apparatus, one of its functions is to respond appropriately to the effects of other systems. So in these cases, there simply is not any malfunction.

Sexual selection can also result in diseases that produce no malfunction. In Italy it has been recorded that because men found women with goitres attractive, the incidence of goitres actually increased (Dubos, 1965, p.11)! Sexual selection could easily result in the selection of painful and distressing conditions because they happened to be attractive to the opposite sex. But the fact that a goitre might assume a function would not mean it is not a disease.

The point is most obvious with biological systems that have been given functions by genetic engineering. A malevolent dictator might get his genetic engineers to programme us all with some dreadful hereditary disease for some purpose or other. He might get his engineers to give us all Huntington's chorea. This is a hereditary disease that results in dementia and problems with movement only in the patient's thirties. He might feel that such subjects had expended their economic usefulness, and should be programmed to self-destruct in this way. Such a process would not cause any malfunction, but it would still be a disease.

Of course, it could be objected that although the goitre acquired a function (of attracting males), it also produced other malfunctions (for example, in swallowing and breathing), and for *this* reason is a disease. Similarly, it could be argued that Huntington's chorea achieves its functional effect by causing malfunctions elsewhere. But again, we could imagine a perverse male fascination for women experiencing swallowing or breathing difficulties. And in this way argue that no malfunction at all is produced – the affected systems have *dual* functions.

Being productive of a malfunction is also not necessary for being a disease for the following reason. Organisms have many traits that do not have any function. Some traits like our appendices may have had function in the past. Other traits like our blood groups may have been acquired by genetic drift and not through natural selection. Other traits like our chins may be the product of genes that code for traits that do have functions – our chins are the result of two genes controlling the shape of the jaw which have evolved to give us the mouth space for diction.

It may be that a woman's capacity for orgasm is something that does not have a function, but is the accidental result of the fact that men and women are made out of the same genetic blueprint. Suppose too that some process, say a viral infection, interferes with a woman's capacity for orgasm. Such a process would be very distressing, and I think we would be correct to classify it as a disease. This would be so even though no function would have been disrupted, and so producing a malfunction is not necessary for being a disease.

There is a further reason why it is not a necessary condition. It may be that (in many species) after a certain age an organism can no longer contribute to a person's biological fitness. This may arise because the organism ceases to be capable of reproduction – as in the case of the female menopause. It might be argued that because no contribution can be made to the differential survival of her genotype after the menopause, the female's organs cease to play a causal role in the selection of her traits. And if this is so, her organs cease to have any function. But if they cease to have any function, they cannot malfunction. But if a post-menopausal woman were to get heart failure, she would have a disease even though she has no malfunction.

Of course it might be argued that post-menopausal women *do* continue to play a causal role in the selection of their traits – a mother can care for her children and grandchildren, and thereby continue to exert a causal influence on the selection of her traits. And hence her organs will not cease to have a function when she ceases to be able to reproduce. But although this reply is in principle correct, we can imagine women not making such contributions, and yet we would still want to say that they could become diseased. And no doubt there are organisms that continue to exist after they have made their last contribution to the survival of their genotype. After reproducing, such an organism's organs would cease to have any functions, and hence would not be capable of malfunctioning. But such an organism can still get a disease.

It might be felt that this shows that our concept of function is at fault. It might be argued that parts with functions necessarily serve the organism's good, so that if a part enables a women to achieve happiness, then it has a function. But we have provided independent reasons for thinking that we have given the correct account of our concept of function. Such an account only sounds strange because we mistakenly believe that organs are there for our benefit. And hence we think that even when they have ceased to exert an influence on their selection, they will have a function because they continue to serve our good (by keeping us alive). We soon learn that many functions do not serve our good, and that like the male mite of the genus *Adactylidium*, we are expendable after we have made our contribution to our biological fitness. This unfortunate mite mates with his sisters while still inside his mother, and is born only to die seconds later, having already exhausted his biological role (Gould, 1980, p.73). Such demise does not mean he has developed some organ malfunction – his organs have ceased to have any function now that he has made his full contribution to his biological fitness.

Being productive of a malfunction is not a sufficient condition for being pathological, and in contexts where the cause of the condition is obscure, is not sufficient for being a disease either. Suppose that we did indeed have some self-destruct process that had been naturally selected. Let us suppose that some viral infection, or any other process which did not have an obvious cause, interfered with the self-destruct mechanism. If the mechanism in question were that of ageing, and this process enables us to live to, say 200-years-old, we would not think we had acquired some disease. If it was a viral infection, we would consider it to be a symbiosis, like that between ants and their intestinal protozoa that enable them to digest wood. We have argued that being a process productive of a malfunction should be a sufficient condition for being a disease in contexts where the condition in question does not have an obvious explanation. But it is not. And since such a process is not pathological, being productive of a malfunction is not sufficient for being pathological.

In summary, then, being a process productive of malfunctioning is not necessary for being a disease. And in contexts where the condition does not have an obvious explanation, being a process productive of a malfunction is not sufficient for being a disease either. Hence we will have to look elsewhere for our account of disease.

Similarly, being a condition that produces a malfunction is not necessary for being a pathological condition. It is not necessary because at least one sort of pathological condition – diseases – need not be processes that produce malfunctioning – interference with a woman's capacity for orgasm will be a pathological condition but not a condition that results in a malfunction. It is not sufficient because there are conditions which produce malfunctions but yet are not pathological conditions (in the form of diseases) – interferences with biological systems that impair the good of the individual (like self-destruct systems) would be productive of a malfunction but would not be pathological conditions. The next task is to see whether the concept of harm can fulfil the role that the concept of malfunctioning failed to do.

# CHAPTER 8
# THE CONCEPT OF HARM

## Introduction

Normativism is the thesis that the concept of disease is value-laden and the most plausible Normativist Theory defines diseases in terms of harm. But in order to assess whether the account of disease in terms of harm is indeed a normative one, we first have to see whether it is true that the concept of harm is a value-laden notion.

It is important to settle the issue of the value-ladenness of the concept of disease. If the concept of disease is a purely descriptive concept, then disagreements as to what is a disease will be easy to settle. To discover whether smoking and hyperactivity are diseases, all we need to do is to discover the value-free facts of the matter. On the other hand, if the concept of harm is value-laden, then whether these conditions are diseases will depend on our values. This means it will be difficult to settle disagreements over classification even among those who share the same concept of disease (unless disagreements are due to mistaken beliefs as to the value-free facts of the matter), but who have different values. And then there seems no way we can prevent the concept of disease being used to enforce the particular values of each culture.

## The logic of harm

When we harm an object, we make it worse off. Thus in order for something to be harmed, it must then have a good or well-being that can be impaired. The logical connection between being harmed and having a good or well-being is supported by the fact that we cannot harm just any object. We cannot harm a stone, faeces, garbage, a catastrophe, and so on. It is only things that have a good or well-being that can be made worse off. Organisms can be harmed because they have a good or well-being.

Some may argue that this is mistaken. One speaks of droughts harming the economy, or terrorist bombings harming the tourist trade, while it is not the case that the economy or the tourist trade has a good or well-being. However, to the extent that it makes sense to talk of some entity flourishing, so it makes sense to talk of that entity being harmed. And it does make sense to talk of the economy or tourist trade flourishing. Because the paradigm sort of thing that flourishes is a living thing, so the paradigm sort of thing that has a good is an organism. Von Wright makes this point:

> The question 'What kinds or species of being have a good?' is therefore broadly identical with the question 'What kind or species of being have a life?' And one could say that it is *metaphorical* to speak of the good of a being, to the same extent as it is metaphorical to speak of the life of that being (von Wright, 1963, p.45).

In order then to understand the concept of human harm, we must give an account of what constitutes human good or welfare.

The notion of 'being worse off' implies the existence of a relationship between two states:

> Someone in state S has been harmed if and only if he is worse off in state S than he would otherwise have been.

To claim that someone has been harmed is to claim that the relationship of being worse off exists between the individual's present state and the state he would have been in.

This might seem problematic because it generates the Epicurean problem: How can we show that death is harmful? Epicureans used to say: 'Where he was, death was not, and where death was, he was not.' They argued that death is not harmful because there is no one who at one time is well off, and who at a later time becomes worse off. When one is alive, one has not been harmed by death. But when one is dead, one has ceased to exist, and hence there is no one existing to be in a worse off state. So there is no one who has been made worse off. And hence death does no harm.

We can avoid this absurdity if we assume that an individual's non-existence is a particular sort of state of that individual. It might be objected that it is not a state of the individual because with all other states, the individual must exist in order to be in these states.

135

But this is not so for the state of non-existence. But all this shows is that non-existence is a peculiar sort of state – it does not prove that it is not a state at all. For our purposes, I will assume that the non-existence of the individual is a (peculiar) state of that individual.

A distinction seems necessary between being harmed on balance or overall, and being harmed in some way. Joe takes amino-glycoside antibiotics for a life-threatening infection. The antibiotics save his life – had he not taken them, he would have died. But unfortunately, they make him deaf. It seems that we want to say that the antibiotics did not harm him overall – he is better off being alive and deaf than being dead. Nevertheless, we want to say that the antibiotics did Joe *some* harm by making him deaf. But if we define the notion of 'some harm' as above, we will have to conclude that the antibiotic does Joe no harm. This is because it is not the case that it makes Joe worse off than he would otherwise have been, for he is better off with his deafness than he would be if he were dead! It seems that the above definition only gives an account of 'overall harm'.

It might seem plausible to give an account of 'some harm' in the following way:

> Someone in state S has received some harm if and only if
> there is some respect R in which he is worse off in state S
> than he would otherwise have been.

The idea is that the antibiotic did Joe some harm because in respect of his hearing, he is worse off than he would otherwise have been. But in our example, this is simply not the case. If Joe had not taken the antibiotics, he would also not have been able to hear, because he would have been dead! Therefore, in respect of his hearing, he is *not* worse off than he would otherwise have been!

While we accept that the antibiotic did not harm Joe overall, we still feel that Joe has received some harm. This is partly because Joe is now worse off than he was before he took the antibiotics. This suggests we define 'some harm' in this way:

> Someone in state S has received some harm if and only if he
> is worse off in state S than he was before he was in state S.

If we define 'some harm' in this way, we arrive at the following paradox: It is reasonable to assume that in order to be harmed overall, one must have received some harm (which also happens to outweigh any benefits). Fred is about to undergo his pubertal growth spurt, and acquire new physical and emotional powers. Unfortunately, he acquires atrophy of the testicles, and does not acquire these powers. We want to be able to say that the testicular atrophy harmed Fred – he is worse off with the atrophy than he would otherwise have been. But it is not the case that Fred is worse off than he was before the atrophy, because he did not first acquire the new powers and then lose them. And so we are forced (on this account of 'some harm') to conclude that the testicular atrophy did Fred no harm (though harming him overall)!

To solve these problems we have to view the notion of 'some harm' as analogous to any theoretical term in science – it is invoked because of its explanatory power. Judgments of overall harm come first, and these are explained by postulating the existence of components of harm. We first compare total states with total states. We conclude that Joe has not been harmed overall by the antibiotic (because his total present state of being alive and deaf is better than the state of being dead in which he would have been). Nevertheless, he is worse off than he was (because his total present state of being alive and deaf is worse than the total past state of being alive and able to hear). To explain this, we invoke the notion of 'some harm' – the antibiotic did him some harm by making him deaf, but did not harm him overall because it also benefited him (to a greater extent) by saving his life.

Similarly, Fred has been harmed overall by the testicular atrophy – his total present state is worse than the total state he would have been in had he undergone puberty. In order to explain this, we invoke the notion of 'some harm' – the testicular atrophy did him some harm by preventing him acquiring his powers, and this harm outweighed any benefit (for example, of preserving his good soprano singing voice). Judgments of overall harm come first, and the notion of 'some harm' is invoked to explain how this is generated by different components of benefit and harm.

Let us now proceed to give an account of the different theories of human good or welfare, and assess which captures the content of our notion of harm.

### Theories of human good

There are two different sorts of theory providing content to the notion of human good – Naturalist theories (theories that define man's good purely in descriptive terms), and Normativist Theories (theories that define man's good in evaluative terms). What I will show is that the notion of human good (and hence harm) is a normative notion, and hence that any account of the concept of disease in terms of the concept of harm will be a value-laden account. Naturalist theories do not work because they fail to recognize that the notion of being worse off is an evaluative one – some reference to the good or worthwhile life is essential for any account to be correct.

For Naturalists, being harmed consists in a certain sort of fact. They argue that it is a *fact* and not simply a value judgment that strokes, heart attacks and multiple sclerosis are harmful. These judgments do indeed seem to be true, and if this is the case, then it is a *fact* that they are harmful, and not a matter of a value judgment. Each Naturalist theory gives a different reading of what this fact consists in. Let us examine whether any one theory is correct.

Naturalist theories

### (1) The functioning properly theory

On this theory, our good is defined in terms of our proper functioning. But we have seen it is a mistake to identify our good with our functioning properly. The female octopus functions properly when she self-destructs, but her good can hardly be identified with her demise! Similarly, the male praying mantis functions properly in sex without his head, but his good does not lie in the (passionate) loss of his head! Finally, if ageing is a self-destruct mechanism with the function of keeping the population numbers down, we would be functioning properly by gradually losing our powers and dying, but our individual good or welfare would not consist in this slow demise.

On this Naturalist theory, being harmed consists in the fact of acquiring a malfunction. A stroke is harmful because it induces a malfunction, and the fact that it is harmful consists in this fact. But if being harmed consists in a fact, it does not consist in the fact that one is made to malfunction. Being a malfunction is not sufficient for being harmed because interference with any of the above self-destruct functions would count as a malfunction, but the organism would not be harmed. Being a malfunction is not necessary because a woman's capacity for orgasm might not have a function, but she would be worse off if something interfered with this ability.

What this shows is that our good cannot be identified with the realization of our (discoverable) nature. If we have any discoverable nature at all, it is a biological nature – if we are anything, we are living organisms. And as Richard Dawkins so eloquently put it, if organisms are anything, they are 'gene machines'. But we have seen that our good does not consist in our being perfect 'gene machines'. For this often means impairing our well-being in the interests of the survival of our genotype.

Evolution has been pretty smart. It has generally ensured that those activities that enhance the survival of our genotype – sex, eating, and so on – are all pleasurable. But it may be in our nature to want what does not serve our good. For example, it might be in the human male's nature to have a desire to the promiscuous, for this is a good way to ensure that he leaves many offspring behind. However, such a desire might not serve his good – it might prevent him from being able to form an intimate and rewarding relationship with one member of the opposite sex which is more fulfilling than having a number of fleeting encounters. Hence he would be better off if he changed his nature in this regard. But if his good is served by changing his nature, then it cannot be identified with his nature.

Our good or well-being cannot be understood in terms of the satisfaction of our biological needs either. Let me define a biological need in the following way:

X has a biological need for N if and only if N is causally necessary for the proper functioning of X.

This account of needs has a number of virtues. Firstly, it is able to explain why any organism needs vitamins, water, food, etc. This is because it malfunctions without them. Secondly, it is able to differentiate between needs and luxuries. We make a distinction between those things that we need, and those things that would simply make us better off. We need protein, but it is not the case that we need caviare. We need water, but we do not need a superdrug that makes us more powerful and intelligent.

On this theory, one is harmed if and only if one's biological needs have been frustrated. But the satisfaction of our biological needs has only a contingent connection to our good. And so this account of harm fails – if being harmed consists in some fact, it does not consist in the fact that one's needs have been frustrated. It fails to provide necessary conditions for being harmed – a woman's capacity for orgasm might not have a function, but it might be causally dependent on substance S. A need for S would not be a biological need, but a woman would be worse off if she lacked S.

It does not provide sufficient conditions either. Suppose our ageing self-destruct mechanism requires the substance G for its proper functioning. We would then have a biological need for G, but we certainly are not worse off if we lack G. And hence we cannot understand the notion of being harmed in terms of the frustration of biological needs.

In fact, we usually operate with a different concept of need. In terms of this concept, a woman has a need for S because she is worse off without it. Similarly, we need G like we need a hole in the head! This is because we are worse off taking G. But this concept of need is understood in terms of the concept of our good or welfare, and hence we cannot use it without circularity to provide the concept of harm with some content. If being harmed consists in some fact, it does not consist in the fact that our biological needs have not been satisfied.

## (2) The hedonistic theory

On this account, man's good consists in his experience of pleasurable mental states and the avoidance of unpleasurable ones. He is harmed only if his experience of pleasure and the avoidance of pain is frustrated. On this theory, what is important is being in certain mental states, and avoiding others. But such a theory seems mistaken.

Suppose there is a viral infection of the brain that induces intense euphoria. However, it also causes dementia – the loss of intellectual faculties, reducing the affected individual to an idiot. Let us call the condition Euphoric Dementia. Suppose too that although reduced to idiocy, the affected individual is able to satisfy his basic biological needs, and so does not have his life expectancy shortened significantly. On the other hand, it produces a mental state that is more pleasurable than any other.

However, few except the most hardened hedonist would see our good as being served by euphoric dementia. Such a condition might make us (subjectively) happy, but would reduce us to contented idiots, and would be regarded as a misfortune by most. As Thomas Nagel argues:

> Suppose an intelligent person receives a brain injury that reduces him to the mental condition of a contented infant, and that such desires as remain to him can be satisfied by a custodian, so that he is free from care. Such a development would be widely regarded as a severe misfortune, not only for his friends and relations, or for society, but also, and primarily, for the person himself (Nagel, 1979, p.9).

On this Naturalist theory, the fact of being harmed consists in the fact that one is deprived of pleasure or subjected to pain. A stroke is harmful because becoming paralysed deprives one of many pleasures. But if being harmed consists in some fact, it does not consist in this sort of fact.

Being made less able to avoid pain and attain pleasure is not necessary for being harmed – we are harmed by Euphoric Dementia even though it promotes rather than frustrates our experience of pleasurable states. Our good does not consist in just being in a certain mental state. It also consists of our exercising certain powers, and achieving certain goals through our actions.

It is not sufficient for being harmed either. It is known that if electrodes are inserted into the pleasure centres of any mammal, they learn to stimulate their pleasure centres to the exclusion of anything else. So much so that laboratory rats have been known to die from exhaustion, hunger and thirst in their frantic pursuit of pleasure. There is no reason to believe that we would behave any differently. However, if we are given such a facility of stimulating our pleasure centres, we would fast become passive, albeit content, vegetables. By removing such an implant, we would make ourselves less able to attain pleasure, but we would not be thereby harming ourselves. And hence being made less able to achieve pleasure is not sufficient for being harmed.

It might be objected that this theory fails not because hedonism is mistaken, but because it is a mistaken account of hedonism. As Derek Parfit remarks:

*Narrow Hedonists* assume, falsely, that pleasure and pain are two distinctive kinds of experience. Compare the pleasures of satisfying an intense thirst or lust, listening to music, solving an intellectual problem, reading a tragedy, and knowing that one's child is happy. These various experiences do not contain any distinctive common quality. What pains and pleasures have in common are their relations to our desires. On the use of 'pain' which has rational and moral significance, all pains are when experienced unwanted, and a pain is worse or greater the more it is unwanted. Similarly, all pleasures are when experienced wanted, and they are better or greater the more they are wanted. These are the claims of *Preference Hedonism* (Parfit, 1984, p.493).

According to 'narrow hedonism', one is worse off without Euphoric Dementia, but on 'preference hedonism', if one prefers being lucid and unhappy to being demented and euphoric, then one is not better off with the dementing condition. Thus preference hedonism is able to avoid this objection.

Similarly, towards the end of his life, Freud was suffering from cancer of the larynx, and was in a great deal of pain. But he refused to take sedating pain-killers because he preferred being lucid but in pain to being pain-free but stuperous. On narrow hedonism, we are forced to say that Freud was worse off without the drugs, which is not what we would want to say. But on preference hedonism, we can say that he was better off without the drugs.

However, imagine there is a tumour of nervous tissue that operates exactly like Robert Nozick's experience machine – it manufactures well-orchestrated hallucinations in all sensory modalities in answer to all our strongest desires (Nozick, 1974, p.42). If we most want to climb Everest, the tumour gives us the experience we would have were we actually to climb Everest. Let us call this condition Tumour Hallucinans. Whatever we most want to do, the tumour gives us the experience we would have if such desires were fulfilled. In addition, it ensures that we are never the wiser for being deceived – it also induces the conviction that such experiences are veridical.

On preference hedonism, we would all be better off if we acquired Tumour Hallucinans. But few of us would see our good as consisting in acquiring such a condition – our good in some way consists of our *living* our lives, and not having them lived for us by the tumour. Hence we cannot give an account of our good or welfare in terms of subjective mental states alone. If being harmed consists in some fact, it does not consist in the fact of being made less able to experience pleasure and avoid pain.

## (3) The desire-satisfaction theory

On this theory, our good is seen to consist in the satisfaction of our interests, as understood as being derived in some way from desires. We are harmed if and only if our interests (as understood in terms of desires) are frustrated. Whether this theory is correct depends on how we understand the notion of interests, and in this section I will argue that a definition of interests in terms of desires fails to capture the notion of human good – we will have to rely on a normative conception of interests for this.

This theory is not equivalent to preference hedonism. According to preference hedonism, it is only mental states that can make us better or worse off. On preference hedonism one is not made worse off by Tumour Hallucinans because it generates all the experiences one most wants. But on this theory, if actually doing something (rather than having the experience of doing it) is what one wants, then one *is* made worse off by the tumour. Thus, if what one most wants is actually to climb Everest, and not simply to have the illusion of climbing Everest, then one's good will not be served by Tumour Hallucinans. And hence the theories are distinct.

We must be careful to distinguish between one of Jake's interests, and Jake's best or overall interests. Smoking might be one of Jake's interests, but is not in his best interests because it will frustrate other more numerous and weightier interests – such as his interest in living a long life. On this theory, Jake's best interests are constructed out of his individual interests.

Brian Barry contrasts want-regarding (Naturalist) theories of interest with ideal-regarding (Normativist) theories – a theory of interests is want-regarding if and only if interests are derived from desires (present or future) without reference to what ought to be desired (Barry, 1965, p.40). Such a theory will give an account of human good or welfare in terms of the satisfaction of desires. Richard Hare is an exponent of a want-regarding (Naturalist) account:

To harm somebody is to act against his interests. What then are

143

his interests? It is fairly obvious that the notion of interests is tied in some way or another to the notion of desires and that of wanting. Admittedly, it is not universally the case that if we want something, it is in our interest to have it, nor that if something is in our interest, we want it. ... I hope it may be granted that there is some ... connection ... between the notions. That there is, is evident from the fact that it would be scarcely intelligible to claim that a certain thing was in a man's interest, although he neither wanted it, nor had ever wanted it, nor would ever want it, nor anything that it was a necessary or sufficient means to, nor might any of these things be the case (Hare, 1972, p.97).

To evaluate the claim that interests are to be understood in terms of desires, let us see just how a Naturalist theory might construct interests from wants.

Percy wants a drink from the well. But he has no interest in drinking from the well because, unbeknown to him, the well is poisoned. The Ignorance Amendment avoids this problem – Percy has no interest in drinking from the well because this is not what he would want if he were not ignorant. If interests are derived from desires that do not depend on mistaken beliefs or reasoning (what we might call enlightened desires), we can avoid his objection.

A has an interest in X if and only if it satisfies some enlightened desire of A.

James is filled with ennui and does not want to go punting, even though he knows he will enjoy it. James has an interest in joining his friends even though he does not have a present desire to do so. The Possible Future Desires Amendment avoids this problem – once James is out with his friends, he will acquire the desire to go punting which he can then satisfy. It is because joining his friends will satisfy some possible future desire that James has an interest in joining his friends:

A has an interest in X if and only if it satisfies some present or possible future enlightened desire of A.

This amendment also enables the theory to solve the problem of those who discount the future. Marmaduke has an interest in going shopping now even though he does not have any present desire to eat or to avoid future hunger. He has this interest because he will come to have a desire for food which he will then be in a position to satisfy if he goes shopping now.

Note that we cannot avoid the problem of moods by arguing that James has an interest in going punting because this is what he would want if he were not in that mood of ennui. If Gertrude does not want to commit suicide because she is in an optimistic mood (and is no longer depressed), we would have to infer by parity of argument that she has an interest to commit suicide, because this is what she would want if she were not in her optimistic mood!

If human good is to be derived from desires, the class of desires will have to be restricted by the Self-regarding Amendment. This amendment is also needed to make self-sacrifice or altruism logically possible. If we accept that those who perform acts of self-sacrifice by giving up their lives to save their children, or by giving up their health down a coal-mine to support their children, are motivated by a desire that outweighs other desires, we seem forced to say that it is in their (best) interests to sacrifice themselves – that their good or welfare consists in their death or ill health, and also that they are not being altruistic. But this is absurd.

We can make this case stronger by changing the story – suppose the man to sacrifice himself for his children is told that he can be hypnotized to forget that he ever had children, and go on to lead a happy life after they are dead. However, even with this information, he might most want to save his children. Here it seems clear that *his* good or welfare consists in not sacrificing himself – but we cannot say this on this account of interests and human good. Although his strongest interest lies in saving the children, *his* welfare does not lie in this direction (Hubin, 1980, p.75).

To avoid this problem, a person's good or welfare must be derived from a certain class of interests – namely, self-regarding interests. Self-regarding interests are interests derived from self-regarding desires. And self-regarding desires are desires for states of affairs where the self has certain properties or stands in certain relations (Williams, 1973, p.263). If I have a desire to be happy, this is a self-regarding desire because I desire that I have the property of being happy. If I desire your happiness, this is an other-regarding desire because I desire that you have the property of being happy. This latter desire is not for any state of affairs where I have any properties or stand in any relations.

On the other hand, if I want to make you happy, this is a self-regarding desire because it is not simply a desire for your happiness, but for a state of affairs, where *I* make you happy. We are not inclined to view such desires as selfless – they are not satisfied by someone else's happiness independently of the self. And this supports the intuition that such desires are self-regarding, even though they are also directed in part at another's happiness.

Someone's desire to save his children is not self-regarding because it is a desire for a state of affairs where his children exist. If however his desire was for *him* to save his children and not for his children to be saved by anybody, this *would* turn out to be a self-regarding interest. And I think this is correct – it is a selfish desire not to want one's children to survive if one has not been instrumental in achieving this. This supports our judgment that a mother who is more concerned with being a good mother than with her children even though she may on the surface be acting selflessly, is in fact acting selfishly.

By deriving a person's good or welfare from this class of desires, we can show that self-sacrifice and altruism *are* possible. This also means that an altruistic or self-sacrificing man's good does not consist in his death:

A has an interest in X if and only if it satisfies some present or possible future enlightened self-regarding desire of A.

Armed with this account so far, one can give an account of what it is to be one's best interests. Gustaff is wondering whether he should preserve his singing voice by castrating himself. He has a desire to sing, and will continue to have this desire, but it is not in his (best) interests to become a castrato. This is because by castrating himself he will frustrate more powerful and more numerous future desires, such as for sex and children. The Maximal Desire-Satisfaction Amendment avoids this problem – it is in Gustaff's (overall) interest not to castrate himself because he will thereby promote the maximal satisfaction of his present and possible future enlightened desires:

X is in A's (best) interest if and only if X promotes the maximal satisfaction of the present and possible future self-regarding enlightened desires of A.

However, imagine being plugged into Jonathan Glover's Horror Machine (Glover, 1984, p.167). This machine gives plugged-in subjects awful experiences, thereby giving them powerful desires to rid themselves of these experiences, which it then satisfies by terminating the experiences. Plugging into the machine will lead to more (numerous and powerful) desires being satisfied than any alternative life, but we would not want to conclude that our good or welfare is served by plugging in!

This objection can be avoided if we distinguish positive and negative desires. Positive desires are desires which we want to have, such as the desire for sexual satisfaction (unless one is a monk!), while negative desires are desires we prefer to be without, like the desire to be free of a present pain (unless one is a masochist!). I want to have the desire for sex, whereas I prefer not to have the desire to be free of pain – I would rather be without the pain that prompts that desire. Now one could argue that although one's good is served by the satisfaction of negative desires (one is better off satisfying one's desire to be free of pain than not satisfying it), one's good is even better served if one is free of the negative desire itself (one is even better off free of the pain that prompted that desire).

Thus one could argue that one's good is not promoted by the acquisition of new powerful negative desires. It would be even better promoted by avoiding such desires altogether. This means our best interests will have to be defined thus:

X is in A's (best) interests if and only if it promotes the maximal satisfaction of present or possible future enlightened self-regarding desires of A (with the proviso that A's interests are better served by avoiding negative desires than by acquiring and then satisfying them).

The desire-satisfaction theory cannot appeal to the really wants amendment. On this amendment, if the theory generates an implausible consequence, we conclude simply that this was not what the agent really wanted. For example, if an agent persists in wanting to become addicted to heroin in the face of all the relevant information, we might be tempted to conclude that it is not in his interest to do so, because this is not what he really wants.

However, the problem lies in defining 'really wants'. If it is defined in terms of what gives us most pleasure, and what make us feel happy, the theory reduces to hedonism. On the other hand, if it is interpreted in terms of what promotes the good or worthwhile life, the theory ceases to be a Naturalist account, for it has to resort to values in order to generate the right consequences.

The desire-satisfaction theory also cannot avail itself of the rational desire amendment. According to this move, if the theory generates awkward consequences, it can simply conclude that the offending desire was not rational. So we can say of a would-be heroin addict that it is not in his (best) interests to become an addict because this desire is not rational.

Again the problem is exactly how 'rational desire' is to be defined. There are broadly two concepts of rationality. On the formal or means–ends concept, some action is rational if and only if it is the best means to a given end. On this theory, ends are neither rational nor irrational. But if ends or desires themselves are neither rational nor irrational, then we cannot use this concept or rationality to save the theory.

On the substantive concept of rationality, ends or desires can be judged rational or irrational. A desire for self-mutilation, for example, is often considered a paradigmatic irrational desire. However, the problem arises as to how to judge when a desire is irrational. If a desire is irrational when it produces pain or suffering, then the theory again reduces to hedonism. However, if a desire is irrational when it impairs the good or well-being of the individual, then the theory ceases to be a Naturalist one, and requires a reference to values to generate the right consequences.

Richard Brandt employs a cognitive psychotherapy account of a rational desire, and argues that a desire is rational when it survives cognitive psychotherapy (Brandt, 1979, p.113). Or to put it in less grandiose terms, if the desire survives repeated exposure to the facts, it is a rational desire. Thus one might consider the desire to kill all the Russians an irrational desire because it is based on the false belief that all Russians are evil people. If a person with such a desire is exposed to the fact that they are not, the desire will not survive. And hence it is classifiable as an irrational desire.

But will this help? One hopes that our addict ceases to want to be an addict when exposed repeatedly to the facts about the suffering of addiction. In which case we could say that his good did not lie in the satisfaction of such an irrational desire. However, there is no guarantee that when the facts have been repeatedly examined, the person will desire what serves his own good.

In addition, it might be that our most important desires, for example, our desire to achieve something worthwhile, would not survive the repeated examination of the fact that we are specks of cosmic dust. This 'cognitive psychotherapy' might make us apathetic, and fill us with a sense of futility. But it would be wrong to conclude that desires defeated in this way are irrational, and even more misguided to think that we would be better off getting rid of them. Our good is better served by living a life full of purpose rather than full of apathy. So this account of rationality will not do the trick either.

Similarly, our desire to do anything at all might be sustained by the belief that we are free agents. However, this belief might not survive the repeated examination of the scientific facts (and philosophic arguments) that support determinism. As a result of all this 'cognitive psychotherapy', we might again become apathetic, believing that everything is determined and that there is no point bothering to change things. But we might be a lot better off if we continued to believe that there was such a thing as free will.

On this account, then, human good consists in the maximal satisfaction of present and possible future enlightened self-regarding desires. Someone is harmed if and only if we frustrate the satisfaction of his interests (so understood). However, I do not think that this theory will work. I may know that I could acquire a very powerful desire for heroin, but it does not seem correct to say that it is in my (best) interests to take heroin should this desire outweigh other present and possible future desires in strength. This is not just because I might develop counterbalancing desires to avoid the suffering of addiction.

Imagine the powerful Brave New World drug Soma that produces the same euphoria as heroin but with none of its ill-effects. It still seems that our good does not lie in letting ourselves be reduced to a perpetual state of vegetative euphoria. Hence our concept of interests is not want-regarding, and our good or well-being cannot be understood in terms of such a notion of interests, that is, in terms of the satisfaction of desire.

Thus it follows that if being harmed consists in a fact, it does not consist in the fact of having one's desires thwarted. The desire-satisfaction theory does not provide necessary conditions for being harmed – we are harmed if we are reduced to a state of vegetative euphoria even though this is what we most want. Becoming an addict might generate the most powerful possible set of desires which I could then go on to satisfy. But my good does not lie in becoming an addict.

149

The theory does not provide sufficient conditions either. Imagine there is a form of dementia called Monomaniacal Dementia. The affected individual acquires a powerful desire to do something trivial, like a desire to play tiddly-winks all day, or a desire to build towers of bottletops all day, as well as a desire to have this desire. It seems implausible to argue that should this desire outweigh in strength all the individual's other present and possible future desires (taken together), that his good is served by acquiring Monomaniacal Dementia.

The theory also falls foul of Derek Parfit's Repugnant Conclusion (Parfit, 1984, p.498). Suppose that I could either have a life of 50 years where my major desires are satisfied, or a life in which only my minor desires are satisfied, but which is long enough such that total desire satisfaction of this life outweighs that in the first life. My good would not be served by leading a life that was barely worth living, but which was long enough so that the amount of desire-satisfaction exceeded that achieved in a short but satisfying life. My welfare would be better served by leading the shorter but satisfying life. But this is not something that is entailed by the desire-satisfaction theory. Therefore, if being harmed consists in any fact, it does not consist in the fact that desires have been frustrated.

### The Normative Theory

I think that we can avoid the problems facing the previous theories if we adopt a Normative view of man's good and well-being. On this theory, our good or welfare is constructed from ideal-regarding interests. We have an interest in just those things that we judge will enable us to lead a good or worthwhile life. Thus we judge that we do not have an interest in acquiring Euphoric Dementia, or Tumour Hallucinans, or becoming an addict, or acquiring Monomaniacal Dementia, etc. This is because we do not consider that such lives are worth living, and so we do not judge that we have an interest in such things.

On this theory too, someone is worse off, if and only if, his interests are impaired. But here someone's interests are impaired if and only if, his leading a good or worthwhile life is interfered with. This is not of course to say that if one has some disease or disability that one is not able to lead a good or worthwhile life – on the contrary, it is often such conditions that spur us on to make something of our lives. It is just that we have a better chance of leading a rich and full life if we are free from disease or disability.

This theory is distinct from the desire-satisfaction theory. Suppose that I am captured by neo-Nazis, and brainwashed into desiring the extermination of non-Aryan races. On the desire-satisfaction theory, my good lies in the satisfaction of these defective values. But on the Normative theory, my good does not lie in what I know is not a worthwhile life. Thus the two theories are distinct.

It is difficult to give a characterization of what the good or worthwhile life consists in, but it is not difficult to give an account of what it is that will make us worse off, that is, harm us. This is because many human powers are needed for *any* conception of the good life. It is difficult, although not impossible, to conceive of a good life needing focomelia, or absent limbs. Or to conceive of a good life needing paralysis, or blindness. And so on. This means it is easier to give a characterization of what makes someone worse off than it is to say what it is that makes someone better off.

But I would like to make some points. Firstly, there is not just *one* sort of worthwhile life – a worthwhile life might consist in people realizing their different worthwhile potentials, and so for one person it will consist in the contemplative life, and for another in a life of action. In this sense, one man's meat may be another man's poison – what makes one worse off may make another better off. A condition increasing the concentration of endurance muscle fibres would promote the good of a long distance runner, but impair the good of a sprinter.

Secondly, it is difficult to think that a life would be worthwhile unless one had a positive desire for it. This is not a matter of conceptual necessity, for someone could always argue that one's good or welfare lay in serving God, even if one did not want to. And he would not be talking nonsense. Nevertheless, most of us think that in order for a life to be worthwhile, it must be desired for its own sake.

Thirdly, the worthwhile life *does* seem to have something to do with the satisfaction of desires, and the achievement of happiness. Perhaps the best way to put it is this: A person's good or welfare consists in the satisfaction of worthwhile desires and the enjoyment of worthwhile pleasures. The Normative theory of our good or well-being does not see the satisfaction of desire simpliciter, or the achievement of pleasurable states of mind simpliciter, as constituting man's good. It sees man's good as only enhanced by the satisfaction of *worthwhile* desires and pleasures.

Most importantly for our purposes, we have seen that the concept of harm is a Normative one. This is further supported by the fact that all the Naturalist theories examined failed to give an account of human good and harm precisely because they did not recognize the evaluative dimension to the concept. Harm only consists in the malfunction of systems worth having, or the frustration of worthwhile pleasures, or the frustration of worthwhile desires. This constitutes a powerful argument that it is only when an account recognizes the evaluative dimension that it will succeed. Obviously, I might not have looked hard enough for a Naturalist theory that captures our concept of harm, but it is difficult to see how it could succeed.

We have seen that the only amendments that saved the Naturalist theories were ones that made references to the good or worthwhile life. This too is evidence that the correct theory will be a Normative one. For example, the rational desire amendment of the desire-satisfaction theory only saves the theory at the expense of defining rational desires in terms of what serves our good or welfare. Similarly the Really Wants Amendment saves the theory only at the expense of defining real desires in terms of those aimed at our good or well-being.

There is further evidence that the concept of harm is normative. This comes from the fact that different people's values lead to different things being considered harmful. This can be best explained by adopting that Normativist theory, which assumes that the concept of harm (and welfare) is value-laden. When the Naturalist theories are viewed as providing different accounts of the good or worthwhile life, we can see how it is possible for there to be genuine disagreements. For example, the hedonist considers that we are better off with the dementing euphoria because he sees the good life as consisting in pleasurable experiences, and we disagree because we do not. So whether the condition of dementing euphoria is considered harmful or not seems to depend on what values are held by those judging the condition.

Similarly, we can explain disagreements over whether disruption of the functioning of some faculty makes us better or worse off. Suppose there is a condition that disrupts the functioning of the repressing mechanism that shields us from painful truths. The (narrow) hedonist would see such a condition as impairing our well-being, and would judge that we are worse off because of it. On the other hand, the existentialist would see such a condition as promoting our good, because he sees the worthwhile life as the authentic existence, and so we are better off without it. It is because the notion of being worse off is normative or evaluative that such conflicts can arise.

In conclusion, the concept of being worse off is a normative notion, and cannot be understood in terms of such descriptive notions as the concepts of malfunction, biological needs, pleasure, and desires. Being harmed does not consist in some complex fact – the concept of harm is a normative notion:

X does A some harm if and only if X makes A less able to lead a good or worthwhile life.

It is time to see whether this account of harm can be used to understand the concept of disease.

# CHAPTER 9
# THE NORMATIVIST THEORY

## Introduction

In this chapter I will explore the Normativist thesis that the concept of disease is value-laden, and is to be understood in terms of the value-laden notion of harm. I have shown that the concept of harm is an evaluative one – judging that some condition makes us worse off (that is, harms us) is to judge that it interferes with the living of a good or worthwhile life.

Many philosophers argue that the concept of disease is a normative or evaluative notion. William Goosens is one:

> Categories mediating the interaction between patient and doctor, like 'disease', 'injury', 'sick', and 'health', do not make functional sense unless there is some connection to benefit [making us better off] and harm [making us worse off]. Since medicine naturally responds to pressing needs, most key medical concepts are negative and connect to harm (Goosens, 1980, p.106).

Tristram Engelhardt argues:

> The concept of disease acts not only to describe and explain, but also to enjoin to action. It indicates a state of affairs as undesirable and to be overcome. It is a normative concept; it says what ought not to be. As such, the concept incorporates criteria of evalution, designating certain states of affairs as desirable and others as not so (Engelhardt, 1975, p.127).

Joseph Margolis remarks:

> The important thing is that the concept of illness is distinctly

value-laden in the sense that, however we extend it or whatever adjustments we may make in its criteria and conditions, we are likely to preserve its signifying some departure from acceptable norms of health (Margolis, 1969, p.64).

These accounts agree that the notion of disease is a normative one – being diseased consists in being worse off than some norm of well-being.

I have argued that causing a biological malfunction is neither necessary nor sufficient for being a disease (or pathological). It is not necessary because interference with some non-functional systems count as diseases. It is not sufficient because interference with self-destruct systems with functions do not count as diseases. What explains why these are counterexamples is that these processes either have or lack a connection to harm. The reason why interference with systems without functions count as diseases is that they cause harm. And the reason why interferences with systems with functions do not count as diseases is that they do not cause harm. The Normativist theory succeeds where the Naturalist theory failed, and so we have some reason to believe that the account of disease in terms of the notion of harm is correct.

## Death, disability, discomfort, and disfiguration

We judge that some process is a disease because of the effects this process has on us. There is a number of different classes of effects that determine whether the cause of these effects is to count as a disease (or pathological). If a condition causes death, we are likely to classify the condition as a disease. Ventricular fibrillation is a disease because it causes death. If a condition causes disability, we are likely to classify the condition as a disease. Multiple sclerosis causes disabilities, and is thereby classified as a disease. Conditions causing discomfort are also classified as diseases. Trigeminal neuralgia is a disease because it causes facial pain. If a condition causes disfiguration, we classify it as a disease. Vitiligo or acne is a disease because it is disfiguring.

Charles Culver and Bernard Gert note that many theories have made this point:

Many accounts of disease have linked the concept very closely

> to the suffering of death, pain, or disability, but without
> attempting to draw out the apparently obvious but unexplained
> common feature in death, pain, and disability (Culver and
> Gert, 1982, p.69).

They go on to argue that what death, disability, and discomfort have in common is that they are effects 'that all persons acting rationally will avoid unless they have an adequate reason not to' (Culver and Gert, 1982, p.75). This they take to be the meaning of 'harm', and so conclude that what pain, death, and disability have in common is that they are all harms (or evils).

However, such an account is not illuminating because they simply define rationality in terms of the avoidance (other things being equal) of pain, disability and death. So the account is circular: pain is an evil because it is rational to avoid it (other things being equal), and it is rational to avoid it because it is pain – this is how rationality is to be understood.

What I want to show is that death, disability, discomfort, and disfiguration *do* have something in common, and this is that they are all ways in which we can be made worse off. This is further evidence that the concept of disease is a normative notion. Let us start with the concept of disability.

Only things that make us worse off are disabling. Suppose Simon does not have an appendix. He is thereby unable to get appendicitis, but he is not thereby disabled. This is because such a capacity is not worth having, and Simon is not worse off with this inability. Some individuals are not able to curl their tongues, but we do not consider such a lack a disability because they are not worse off with this inability. It is only where an ability is worth having and we are worse off without it that its absense counts as a disability. This shows that if the concept of disease is connected to the notion of being disabled, it too will be a normative notion.

Being an inability that makes one worse off is only a necessary condition for counting as a disability – not every inability we would be better off without counts as a disability. We are all worse off than we would be if we could fly, but this does not mean we are all disabled. This is because being able to fly is not a *normal* human ability.

Conditions that cause death are ultimately disabling – being alive is necessary for being able to do most things worth doing. By robbing us of these abilities, death makes us worse off. This does not mean that death is necessarily harmful (overall) – if someone has terminal cancer, and is suffering terribly from intractable pain, there is often a good case for arguing that such a person would be better off dead.

It may seem that if the concept of disease is connected to the concept of death, it is not a normative concept. This is because the concept of death is a purely descriptive notion – when we judge that someone is dead, we are not making a value-judgment. We simply describe that his brain is in such a state that it is no longer capable of sustaining consciousness. But the concept of disease is not necessarily connected to the concept of death – it is only when death makes us worse off that a condition causing death is classified as a disease. Let me explain.

If we were immortal, we might classify conditions causing death differently. Suppose immortality is hell, making life tedious and boring, and reducing us to apathetic vegetables (Williams, 1973, pp.82–100). Suppose too that there is a single genetic condition that a few inherit that causes cardiac arrest, and enables those few individuals to die around the age of 200-years-old. The lives of such individuals are not boring, but full of interest and happiness because they are mortal. This condition, in spite of its causing death, is one that would be worth having, and would therefore not be classified as a disease. Whether a condition causing death is harmful (and thereby pathological) depends on whether it is worth having.

Making one worse off is also necessary for something being discomforting. Children who induce vertigo for fun by rolling down hills are not in any discomfort. This is because they are not made worse off by the experience – they enjoy it. On the other hand, the vertigo due to viral labyrinthitis is discomforting because it makes the patients worse off. Whether something causes discomfort depends on whether it makes the person worse off.

It might be objected that if the concept of disease is connected to the concept of pain, it is not normative. This is because the concept of pain is a purely descriptive concept – when we judge that someone is in pain, we do not make a value-judgment. We simply describe the sort of sensation that is being experienced. However, it is only when a condition causing pain makes us worse off that we judge it is a disease. Let me explain.

Suppose we were all masochists, and really enjoyed being in pain – this was something that we spent a great deal of time seeking. Lest it be thought that a sensation not found aversive would not be pain, it must be noted that patients under dissociative anaesthesia and with frontal leucotomies can recognize painful sensations in spite of the fact that they experience no concomitant desire to avoid them – pain is still pain even if not found aversive. As masochists, we would not judge that we would be worse off with a condition like migraine. In such a situation, we would not classify the condition as a disease. And this seems to show that it is only when we judge that pain makes us worse off that a condition causing pain is judged as being a disease.

Similarly, someone is disfigured by some condition only if he is worse off with the condition. A scar is only disfiguring if one judges that one is better off without it. The African tribes that induce patterned scarring do not see such scars as disfiguring because they consider such scars attractive.

Jonathan Barnes points out that if the concept of disease is connected to the concept of disfigurement, it will not be an evaluative notion (Jonathan Barnes in conversation). This is because when we judge that someone is disfigured, we do not necessarily imply he is worse off. Duelling scars disfigured noblemen in the past but did not make them worse off – the scars enhanced their status, and they were better off with them. So it seems that the notion of disfigurement is not an evaluative one.

However, either the noblemen themselves considered the scars disfiguring, or they did not. If they did not, then this example does not challenge the normative nature of the notion (because they are not worse off). If they did, then this too does not undermine the normative nature. They can consider themselves worse off in one respect (their appearance), but better off overall (because improvement of status outweighs the loss of good looks). It is because the distinction between receiving some harm and being harmed overall is ignored that disfigurement is thought of as a descriptive notion. Whether scars are regarded as disfiguring depends on whether we judge that scars make us worse off (in respect of our appearance).

These arguments support the conclusion that the concept of disease is connected to the concept of harm. Conditions causing death, pain, changes in our appearance, or changes in our abilities are only diseases if these consequences make us worse off. It is because we have an interest in being free of pain (and nausea *et al.*), being able to do what we want, and having an attractive physical appearance that conditions such as ventricular fibrillation, trigeminal neuralgia, multiple sclerosis, and vitiligo all make us worse off, and are thereby classified as pathological conditions. Diseases are so classified because they are processes that make us worse off.

## Disease as harm

In this section I will modify and develop the Normativist theory in response to various challenges. A first attempt at a definition of disease in terms of harm might look like this:

A has a disease P if and only if P is a bodily/mental process that harms A.

Note that this is to be understood as: A has a disease P if and only if P is a process that makes A worse off than he would otherwise have been. It would be a mistake to read this as: A has a disease P if and only if P is a process that makes A worse off than he was before he got P. This would mean that there could be no hereditary defects or diseases. Down's syndrome is a disease not because the affected individuals are worse off than they were before they acquired the syndrome – they were never better off, but because they are worse off than they would have been without the syndrome.

This problem is not confined to hereditary conditions. Peter is about to get his pubertal growth spurt, and acquire a whole new range of powers. However, he gets testicular atrophy, and fails to acquire these powers. The testicular atrophy is a disease, but not because it makes Peter worse off than he was before he acquired the condition, because he never first acquired these powers and then lost them. It is a disease because it makes him worse off than he would have been without the condition.

However, we are all worse off at ninety (even if we are healthy) than we are at thirty. We have lost a whole range of powers that we would be better off retaining. So the ageing process is one that makes us worse off than we would have been had we not aged. Nevertheless, ageing is not a disease. There are some people known as non-somniacs who only need an hour of sleep a day (Meddis, 1979, p.123). In spite of the fact that we would be better off if we did not have our normal excessive need for sleep – we could lead two lives – we all do not suffer from a normal form of 'sleeping sickness'! Although there are many (normal) conditions we would be better off without, this does not make us diseased – we are not diseased because we are not Supermen! The definition must therefore be changed:

> A has a disease P if and only if P is a harmful bodily/mental process of an abnormal type.

Because the ageing process and our tendency to sleep for eight hours are normal, in spite of the fact that we would be better off without such processes, they are not diseases.

Not every individual disease of a type will be harmful. Someone with an immune deficiency might be lucky enough never to encounter any pathogenic organisms, and thus never be worse off as a result of this deficiency. Similarly, if a haemophiliac is lucky enough never to be traumatized, he will never suffer as a result of his condition. Nevertheless, these conditions are still diseases. To avoid these counterexamples, the account will have to be modified thus:

> A has a disease P if and only if P is an abnormal bodily/mental process that harms A *in standard circumstances.*

It is because haemophilia and immune deficiency generally make us worse off that they are diseases.

Disease-status is thus a relational notion. Whether some condition is a disease (or pathological) depends on the world which the organism inhabits. In a world filled with useless noise, osteo-sclerosis resulting in deafness would not be a disease, because in these standard circumstances it would not make us worse off. It is because the standard circumstances are different that the condition is a disease.

Just as one environment's disease is another environment's adaptation, so one species' disease will be another species' adaptation. A condition causing malformed wings in members of the mainland species of fly will be a disease. On the other hand, the same condition will be an adaptation in members of the island species of fly (because it prevents them from flying and being swept out to sea). Therefore, we must amend the definition thus:

> A has a disease P if and only if P is an abnormal bodily/
> mental process that harms members of A's species in
> standard circumstances.

It might seem that this definition too is faulty. In areas that were affected by smallpox, it was to everyone's overall advantage to get cow-pox. This is because cow-pox provides protection against the more dangerous smallpox. Nevertheless, we might still feel that cow-pox is a disease. But we should not be tempted to amend the definition thus:

> A has a disease P if and only if P is an abnormal bodily/
> mental process that does members of A's species *some* harm
> in standard circumstances.

This is because of the following problem. Suppose that a new virus infects us and splices its genetic material into our genome, thereby giving us a whole range of new powers – it increases our IQ, it makes us stronger, it heightens our senses, and so on, enabling us to get much more out of life. But suppose too that it also causes a mild myopia. On the above definition the viral infection would be a disease because it did some harm. However the huge benefits are unlikely to make us classify the condition as a disease.

I think that the reason why we are still tempted to classify cow pox as a disease even in circumstances where it does not do us overall harm is because we are seduced by the Essentialist Fallacy. It is because cow-pox is an infection and has the same nature as other diseases, that we think it must be a disease. But we have exposed the Essentialist Fallacy, and when we see that being a disease does not consist in having a particular sort of nature, the need to classify cow-pox as a disease (in this context) evaporates. Thus I think we must continue to define disease in terms of *overall* harm, and not *some* harm.

Certain diseases may not harm all members of a species in standard circumstances. This is because one man's ability is another man's disability. George wants to be a basketball player, and so getting pituitary dwarfism is harmful because he is thereby severely disabled as basketball player. However, Fred wants to be a jockey, and so pituitary dwarfism is supremely enabling as far as he is concerned. One and the same condition adversely affects one person's interests (that is, makes him worse off), while it promotes another's interests (that is, makes him better off).

Or take Jill who has no interest in having children – she (unlike the rest of us) would get no pleasure from them. For her, then, infertility would not count as a disability – on the contrary, she would be liberated from concern over contraception. This means we will have to define disease thus:

A has a disease P if and only if P is an abnormal bodily/ mental process that harms *standard* members of A's species in standard circumstances.

It might be objected that conditions like viral warts or athlete's foot, hardly make us worse off, but yet are still diseases. But it is simply not true that they do not make us worse off. They are mild diseases because they do not make us *significantly* worse off, but they are diseases nevertheless because we would be better off to some extent without them.

It might also be objected that there are some conditions classified as diseases or as pathological conditions that do not make us worse off. For example, in 1901 Gilbert described a condition that led to a mildly elevated serum bilirubin. Because the condition led to jaundice (a sign in many diseases), the condition was classified as a disease, and became known as 'Gilbert's disease'. But the condition does not do any harm. In spite of its name, if it does not make us worse off, then the condition is no different from the inability to curl one's tongue, and hardly a disease at all. At most, it is a healthy variant of the norm. And so it is a mistake to classify the condition as a disease.

Debates often go on in medicine as to whether some condition is a disease or merely a normal variant, and it is their harmful nature that determines their disease-status. For example, the leading article in the *British Medical Journal* of 23 June 1984, is entitled 'Mitral valve prolapse: harbinger of death or variant of normal?' Here it is argued that mitral valve prolapse (as picked up by echo-cardiography) is not a disease but a 'variant of normal' because it is not associated with any harmful consequences like shortness of breath, pain, syncope, and sudden death.

I have argued above that we cannot provide sufficient conditions for diseases. There are some processes, like starvation, drowning, sunburn, and barbiturate poisoning, that are not classified as diseases, but nevertheless satisfy the definition. I argued that it was only in contexts where the cause was not obvious that the process had come to be classified as a disease. Nevertheless, the account does provide necessary conditions for being a disease.

The following account does seem to provide necessary and sufficient conditions for something to be pathological:

> A has a pathological condition C if and only if C is an abnormal bodily/mental condition (not necessarily a process) that harms standard members of A's species in standard circumstances.

Someone might object that an overly large and crooked nose is not a pathological condition. But the reason for this seems obscure. Imagine there is an 'ugly bug' that causes normal noses to become ugly in this way. Is it not reasonable to conclude that, like vitiligo, the process is a disease? But if the process is a disease because of the undesirability of this effect, then why is the nose itself not a pathological defect if it is simply inherited? I would conclude that grossly deformed or ugly features are indeed pathological conditions that merit medical intervention. And this explains why the medical profession has become concerned, and ought to be, with such conditions.

It might be further objected that being extremely cold is both unpleasant and mildly disabling (one's limbs are stiff), but it is not a pathological condition. I suspect that this condition is not regarded as pathological because its correction does not require *medical intervention*. On the other hand, conditions like hypothermia are pathological because they do require such intervention. Being cold is corrected by simply sitting near a heater. On the other hand, hypothermia needs medical supervision for complications like arrythmias, and may need correction by sophisticated medical means like peritoneal lavage with warm saline.

It will be circular to define disease in terms of what requires medical intervention if medical intervention is defined in terms of what is needed to combat disease. However, we can define medical intervention purely enumeratively without reference to the notion of disease – in terms of pharmacological and surgical interventions. The account of pathological conditions (including diseases) must be amended thus:

> A has a pathological condition C if and only if C is an abnormal bodily/mental condition which requires medical

163

intervention and which harms standard members of A's species in standard circumstances.

Let us turn now to see whether these definitions can withstand certain objections.

## Objections

In this section I will examine some general objections to this account of disease. Christopher Boorse raises the following one:

> It is obvious that a disease may be on balance desirable, as with flat feet of a draftee or the mild infection produced by innoculation. It might be suggested in response that diseases must at any rate be prima facie undesirable. The trouble with this suggestion is that it is obscure. Consider the case of a disease that has infertility as its sole important effect. In what sense is infertility prima facie undesirable? Considered in abstraction from the actual effects of reproduction on human beings, it is hard to see how infertility is either desirable or undesirable. Possibly those who see it as 'prima facie' undesirable assume that most people want to be able to have children. But the corollary of this position will be that writers of medical texts must do an empirical survey of human preferences to be sure that a condition is a disease. No such considerations seem to enter into human physiological research, any more than they do into standard biological studies of the diseases of plants and animals (Boorse, 1975, p.53).

However, it is precisely because most of us may be harmed by infertility that infertility is a disease. Because the standard human being is worse off without children, infertility counts as a disease. (In fact, there are few conditions that lead to as much suffering.) In addition, it is hardly an objection that surveys have to be made – how else would any biological research determine the functional norm? Even an exponent of the Naturalist theory has to do 'surveys' as to what functional capacity is typical of any given species.

Christopher Boorse also objects that this account of disease fails to apply to the rest of the biological world:

Biologists who study diseases of fruit flies or sharks need not assume that their health is a good thing for us. On the other hand, there is not much sense in talking about the best interests of, say, a begonia (Boorse, 1975, p.53).

The argument is that plants and other animals can have diseases, but since it is doubtful whether they can have interests, it is doubtful whether the account of disease in terms of (ideal-regarding) interests is correct.

This might seem to show that disease should be understood in terms of the concept of malfunction, because plants and animals can certainly have biological malfunctions. But although plants might not have interests (because they cannot have worthwhile desires and pleasures), we can also give an account of disease in plants or animals in terms of the notion of being made worse off. All organisms have a good or well-being which can either be promoted or impaired. And because of this all organisms can be made worse off. In our case our good or well-being is understood in terms of the satisfaction of our (normative) interests, but this need not be the case for organisms that do not have interests. In their case, their good must be understood differently.

A plant may have a self-destruct mechanism that it has acquired by natural selection – this causes it to become the nutrients for its offspring. Suppose it gets a fungal infection that enables it to live a healthy life for ten times as long. On the malfunction theory, this would be a disease. But I am inclined to think that we are likely to view it as a symbiosis, and this would support an account of plant disease in terms of the plant's good. Thus there is no reason to go over to a malfunction account of disease.

There is the following more serious objection. It might be argued that the condition of having black skin in a white racist society is something that makes those individuals worse off. But it would be wrong to say that the condition is a disease. We might try to avoid this by saying that the individual is not made worse off by his black skin but by the social prejudice acting on that trait. But individuals with albinism are also not made worse off by the fairness of their skins, but by the sun's rays acting on that trait. And albinism is still a disease. Norman Daniels points this problem out:

[W]e must specify the range of environments taken as 'natural' for the purpose of revealing dysfunction. The latter is critical to the second feature of the biomedical model: for example, what range of social roles and environments is included in the natural range? If we allow too much to the social environment, then racially discriminatory environments might make being of the wrong race a disease; if we disallow all socially created environments, then we seem not to be able to call dyslexia a disease (disability) (Daniel, 1981, p.156).

But there is a relevant difference between being black and having dyslexia – it is worth while being able to read easily, but being white is not something that is intrinsically worthwhile. But this point does not seem to help. While it is not worth while being white (*per se*), it is certainly worth while avoiding the deprivation that being black might bring. Just as it is not worth while defecating (*per se*), it is worth while being able to avoid the gross abdominal distension and death that this inability would bring.

However, when we are deciding whether some condition is a disease, we are in effect deciding what sort of people we ought to be. As we saw with the case of grief, it is because we do not want to be the sort of people who do not grieve after any great loss that we do not consider that it is a disease. We take ourselves to be even better off as beings capable of grief. Similarly, when deciding whether male balding is a disease, we might acknowledge that we are better off having hair (women find it more attractive), but we might judge that we do not want to be the sort of people that are concerned with such trivia, and regard ourselves as even better off as beings who are not worried by such matters. And so we would conclude that balding is not a pathological condition.

Thus while it might be true that a black man would be better off white in a racist society, we conclude that we would all be better off as beings who are not governed by prejudice. We want to be beings who are not prejudiced in this way, and so take ourselves to be even better off without the prejudice than without the trait that is being prejudiced against. And so we conclude that being black is not a pathological condition. On the other hand, it is because we *do* want to be the sort of beings who can read that we conclude that dyslexia is a disease.

There is another important objection that the account has to face. Suppose that in the future neurology has made great leaps. It has discovered that all human pursuits are caused by specific neurological states. All golfers have one specific nervous condition, all bookworms another, and so on. Suppose too that it has dis-covered that all criminals have a specific (abnormal) neurological state. Suppose too that in general it is true that crime does not pay – criminals end up being worse off (in jail, for example). While it might be the case that we could alter this neurological state by medical means – we could subject all criminals to frontal lobotomy – it might not be considered *appropriate* to do so. We might not consider it appropriate because we feel that such behaviour is, like golfing, freely chosen, and hence not due to some disease. Only if we feel it is appropriate to use medical means will the condition be considered pathological. It is because we do not consider it appropriate to alter criminal behaviour by medical means that we will not consider the neurological state as pathological.

Because of this argument, we will have to amend the definition thus:

> A has a pathological condition C if and only if C is an
> abnormal bodily/mental condition which requires medical
> intervention and for which medical intervention is
> appropriate, and which harms standard members of A's
> species in standard circumstances.

It might be objected that evaluative judgments cannot be true or false, and hence that the Normativist theory entails that disease judgments cannot be true or false. But (so the objection runs), disease judgments *can* be correct or mistaken. We are correct in judging that TB is a disease, and the South American Indians are mistaken not to regard dyschromic spirochaetosis as a disease.

This objection asssumes that normative or evaluative judgments cannot be true or false, and to settle this issue lies outside the scope of this book. But this much can be said: Whether a condition is or is not a disease depends (in part) on whether that condition is an undesirable departure from some norm (of health). The fact that reference to some norm is essential gives us some reason to believe that judgments about diseases are not true or false. We have argued that this health norm is not something that we can discover, and hence the norm is not true of any independently existing state of affairs. Because of the possibility of universal diseases, the norm need not coincide with the discoverable average state for a species. Whether some condition, like ageing, is normal, and hence not a disease, is something that depends on a *decision* we make, and so not something that can be true or false. If we wished to see ageing as a genetic disease everyone has the misfortune to suffer from, we could.

But, if judgments about the existence of norms are not true or false, and do not reflect any independently existing state of affairs, then it follows that judgments about diseases are not true or false either. When we argue that we are correct to classify TB as a disease, and the South American tribe incorrect to classify dyschromic spirochaetosis as a disease, we are simply further endorsing the adoption of one norm rather than another.

Lastly, it might be objected that Normativism commits us to Relativism. If disease judgments are evaluative, then (so the objection runs) we will be forced to accept that whether something is a disease is relative to one's value system. Robert Kendell seems to make this assumption:

> [T]o accept Sedgwick's argument that the attribution of disease, mental or physical, is fundamentally a social value judgment ... would mean that we could never maintain on medical grounds that x or y *were*, or were not, diseases. We could only argue on social grounds that they *ought*, or ought not, to be *regarded* as diseases. ... [W]e could not criticize Russian psychiatrists for incarcerating sane political dissidents in their beastly asylums [on medical grounds]: they would be perfectly entitled to regard political dissent as a mental illness if, as is probably the case, most of their fellow-citizens disapproved of political dissenters and it happened to be more convenient to deal with them as patients than as criminals. (We could still, as laymen, criticize them on humanitarian or political grounds, but not as doctors on medical grounds) (Kendell, 1976, p.508).

Kendell assumes here that Normativism commits us to Relativism, and since this is an unpalatable consequence, Normativism must be wrong. What I will show is that even if Normativism means that disease judgments cannot be true or false, this does not mean we are committed to Relativism.

To show this, we must distinguish Contextualism from Relativism. Contextualism is true of a domain of discourse when the truth of the sentences varies from one system to the next, because the sentences contain relational terms such that the truth conditions also vary from system to system. Relativism is true of a domain of discourse when the truth of the sentences is held to vary from one system to another even though the truth conditions of the sentences remain the same from one system to the next. Relativism commits one to the thesis that one and the same proposition can be true in one system, and false in another, while Contextualism does not commit one to this thesis.

For example, Contextualism is true of sentences about motion – whether the sentence 'X is moving' is true depends on the frame of reference from which the judgment is being made. This is because motion is a relational notion, and the same sentence does not have the same truth conditions in different systems, and hence does not express the same proposition. 'X is moving-relative-to-A' is true in A and B, and 'X is stationary-relative-to-B' is also true in A and B. And so it is not the case that one and the same *proposition* is true in one system and false in another. Contextualism makes the point that one sentence like 'Smoking grass is illegal' is true in a Hippie belief system, but false in an old-fashioned farmer's system simply because the sentence has a different meaning in the different systems.

Contextualism is also true of propositions about disease. Whether a condition is a disease depends on what sort of organism has the condition, and on the relation of that organism to the environment. Sickle-cell trait is not pathological in malarial areas, but is at high altitudes. Insensitivity to growth hormone is not a disease among pygmies, but is a disease among the Masai. Malformed wings is not pathological among island flies, but is pathological among mainlanders. Dyslexia is not a disease in a pre-literate environment, but it is in a literate one. And so on. We cannot decide whether a judgment about disease-status is true without considering the relation of the condition to the organism, and the relation of the organism to the environment. One organism's disease is another's adaptation, as is one environment's disease another's adaptation.

What can be inferred from this is that the truth or falsity of a sentence 'x is a disease' varies with the sort of organism that has the condition, and with the sort of environment in which that organism lives. This is because the notion of disease is a relational one. The truth or falsity of the sentence could be made invariant if we filled it out into 'x is a disease-for-humans-in-high-altitudes'. Contextualism, then, is not a controversial thesis – the variation of truth-value of the proposition is explained by the variation of truth conditions which results from the relational nature of the attributions.

Relativism, on the other hand, is the thesis that the truth value of a sentence varies with the belief (and value) system that has been adopted. But if one and the same proposition is to be true in one belief system and false in another, the identity conditions for the proposition must be satisfied. But then, as William Newton-Smith points out: '[P]ropositions are individuated in terms of truth conditions. It is just incoherent to suppose that the same proposition could be true in $\Psi$ and false in $\phi$' (Newton-Smith, 1982, pp.107–8). So Relativism seems incoherent for propositions that are individuated by their truth conditions.

However, if evaluative judgments cannot be true or false, then they must be individuated in some other way. And so a modified Relativism might still be true of such propositions. For propositions that are individuated by expressive conditions, Relativism would amount to the idea that it is correct to endorse one thing if you have one attitude, but not correct to endorse the same thing if you have another attitude. Relativism about disease judgments would amount to the idea that it is correct to judge that Euphoric Dementia is a disease from our point of view, and also correct to judge that it is not a disease from the hedonistic point of view.

But Relativism here is also incoherent. If the proposition 'Euphoric Dementia is a disease' is individuated by its expressive conditions, then it would be incoherent to embrace Relativism, for this amounts to both endorsing and condemning one and the same state of affairs. By judging that it is correct that Euphoric Dementia is a disease, one is disvaluing the possession of that condition. But by also judging that it is correct that Euphoric Dementia is not a disease (from another point of view), one is at the same time not disvaluing the condition. But it is incoherent both to disvalue and not to disvalue the same condition. Thus in accepting that there are no truth conditions for disease judgments, we are not committing ourselves to the claim that if we had a different point of view, TB would not be a disease.

In conclusion, then, we have reason to accept the Normativist theory of disease. Disease is to be understood in terms of the evaluative notion of being harmed. It also requires a reference to some norm – not all conditions that we would be better off without are diseases. The Normativist theory commits us to Normativism – the thesis that the concept of disease is value-laden. As Tristram Engelhardt remarks:

Nature does not reflect a natural standard or norm, because nature does nothing – nature does not care for excellence, nor is it concerned for the fate of individuals qua individuals. Health, insofar as it is to indicate anything more than the usual functions or abilities of the members of the species, must involve judgments as to what members of that species should be able to do – that is, must involve our esteeming a particular type of function (Engelhardt, 1976, p.266).

The Normativist theory also commits us to Contextualism, the thesis that the concept of disease is a relational one. However, it does not commit us to the unacceptable thesis of Relativism.

If Normativism is correct, then we do not have an easy solution to the classificatory problems that we started with. This is not an objection to the theory, for it cannot be assumed that there is an easy solution in the first place. Nevertheless, the theory does not entail that we have a *carte blanche* to call anything we do not like a disease! We are not free to call political dissidence a disease because it is due to normal processes. We are not free to classify as diseased anybody that society finds a nuisance, or who does not conform, because such 'neurological states' causing such behaviour do not do the individual any harm. Our concept of disease does impose some limits on what we can legitimately classify as a disease, and if we violate these limits, we simply cease to speak English.

Even if judging that some condition is a disease is a value-judgment, and not true of any objective norm existing in the universe independently of us, this does not mean that we cannot defend our position. Even if disease judgments are normative, this does not mean we cannot oppose the Russian psychiatrists. Just as we are prepared to defend our value-judgment that Hitler was an evil man, so we are similarly prepared to defend our value-judgment that political dissidence is not a disease. Judging that some condition is a disease commits one to stamping it out. And judging that a condition is not a disease commits one to preventing its medical treatment.

# CHAPTER 10

# DISEASE ENTITIES AS NATURAL KINDS

## Introduction

Do we discover the identities and differences among diseases? Is the number of diseases that exist something that we can discover? Or do we invent disease identity and difference by imposing our taxonomy on the world? Is the number we recognize a product of the taxonomy we choose to adopt? The answers to these questions turn on whether disease entities are natural kinds, and this chapter will be devoted to settling this issue. First let me summarize the position so far.

Firstly, we have seen that being a disease does not consist in having a particular sort of explanatory nature. Secondly, being a pathological condition also does not consist in having a particular sort of explanatory nature. Thirdly, in order for a process or condition to qualify as pathological, it must be abnormal. Fourthly, only if an abnormal process or condition makes the organism worse off does it count as pathological. This ensures that the concept of disease is a normative one.

However, all this does not preclude the possibility that specific disease entities, like TB, multiple sclerosis, Down's syndrome, etc., are natural kinds. That is, it is possible that bodily conditions fall into lower-order natural kinds (and even some higher-order natural kinds like viral infections and auto-immune disorders), but not into such higher-order natural kinds as diseases or pathological conditions. Thus the question of whether disease entities are natural kinds remains open.

This will settle the issue of whether TR applies to the medical domain. TR is the thesis that classificatory systems, or taxonomies, can be correct or incorrect. They are correct when they mirror the natural kinds that exist independently of our taxonomies, and they are incorrect when they fail to do so. In order for TR to be true of any domain, two things have to be the case: Firstly, objects in that domain have to fall into natural kinds, and secondly, the terms that pick out such kinds must have a NKS. Should there be no natural kinds, there would be nothing for the taxonomy to mirror. And should the terms not purport to pick out natural kinds, we could not convict the taxonomy of error for having failed to do so.

Because there are no such higher-order natural kinds as diseases and pathological conditions, and because the terms 'disease' and 'pathology' do not have a NKS, TR for the medical domain is false. However, even though we know that TR is not true of the whole taxonomic hierarchy, it might nevertheless be true of the lower orders of the hierarchy. Just as it is reasonable to defend TR in the biological domain for the lower orders of the taxonomic hierarchy – different species constitute different natural kinds – it is less reasonable to argue that TR applies across the board to the higher orders of the hierarchy as well – it is unlikely that all plants share an explanatory nature in virtue of which they constitute a higher-order natural kind. So the question of whether TR applies to the hierarchical level of disease entities is something that still remains open.

Many philosophers of medicine argue that the divisions among diseases are invented and not discovered. Lester King argues:

> We resolve the difficulty only by admitting that we carve out whatever disease patterns we wish in whatever way we desire. ... [A] disease pattern is a class, or niche in a framework. This framework is a means of approaching and organizing crude experience, that is, for dealing with every-day events in the most satisfactory way. These classes will vary in their utility in the handling of experience. What we call a fever is a very broad and inclusive class. There is only one reason why we should not regard fever as a disease entity and that is, such an entity is so broad and inclusive, so general and nondiscriminating, that it lacks utility (King, 1954, p.201).

What is being claimed here is that we do not discover that fever is not a disease entity. Rather, we decide that it is not because it is more useful to regard scarlet fever, malaria, and so on, as disease entities. Similarly, Robert Kendell criticizes the view that there is a determinate number of diseases awaiting discovery:

> To our generation it is self-evident that diseases ... are nothing
> but man made abstractions, inventions justified only by their
> convenience. ... [W]e find it difficult to credit how an earlier
> generation could have talked of diseases being 'discovered' like
> so many golden sovereigns on a beach, or have imagined that
> there were a finite number of them waiting to be identified
> (Kendell, 1975, p.21).

I will first examine whether disease entities fall into natural
kinds. I will then go on to examine whether it follows from this that
there is a determinate number of disease entities existing independently of us and awaiting enumeration. I will assume that
disease-status has already been settled – we have classified
conditions into diseases (or pathological conditions) and non-
diseases (or normal conditions). The task then is to see whether the
conditions already recognized as diseases fall into natural kinds. In
this way we will discover what constitutes disease identity. I will
investigate whether membership to the same natural kind is
necessary and sufficient for being the same disease entity.

## Are disease entities natural kinds?

What is it for diseases to be natural kinds? Objects fall into a
(complex) natural kind if they share the same nature which explains
their cluster of properties in the same way. For members to
constitute a distinct natural kind, they must have a nature that is
distinct (varies in kind or discontinuously in degree) from members
of different natural kinds. There must be a rarity of intermediate
forms at the level of the explanatory natures if we are to have
distinct natural kinds.

It is not necessary for members of a single natural kind to share
the *same* cluster of properties. For example, ice, water, and steam
all belong to the same natural kind but they do not share the same
cluster of properties. They might share a (narrower) cluster of
chemical properties, but it is not this that makes them members of
the same natural kind. It is because they all consist of molecules of
$H_2O$ that they are members of the same natural kind. Similarly,
male and female mallards (and humans) do not share the same
cluster of properties, but they belong to the same natural kind
because they share the same explanatory nature – they all have the
same genetic blueprint.

This point must be qualified, for it is not true that water, ice, and steam all possess exactly the same explanatory nature – if they did, they *would* have the same cluster of properties. Similarly, it is not true that male and female mallards (and humans) have the same explanatory nature – how could we then explain why they are different? In fact, the explanatory nature of water consists of $H_2O$ molecules *bonded together by loose hydrogen bonds*, and the explanatory nature of ice consists of $H_2O$ molecules *bonded together in a crystal lattice*. But although they have different natures at one level that explains why they do not have exactly the same cluster of properties, at another level they do have the same nature – they all consist of $H_2O$ molecules. Similarly, the nature of men and women differs in the sex chromosomes (men have XY, women XX). However, there is a common nature that is shared by both men and women in virtue of which they both belong to the same biological species. (It is this nature that explains why there is a cluster of properties that is shared by both sexes.) Possession of the same cluster is not necessary for membership to the same natural kind.

Neither, or course, is it sufficient. There are many cases where members of different kinds share the same cluster of properties. For example, fool's gold and real gold share a cluster of properties. But they are not members of the same natural kind because the explanatory nature of gold consists of atoms with 79 protons, while the explanatory nature of fool's gold consists of iron pyrites. Similarly, plant species generated by polyploidy are identical morphologically but belong to different species (because they have different numbers of chromosomes ensuring reproductive isolation).

Nevertheless, possession of a distinct cluster of properties is *evidence* that objects belong to a natural kind – most objects that share a significant cluster of properties will also be members of the same natural kind. In either event, whether there are natural kinds, and whether two conditions belong to the same natural kind, are empirical questions, and ones that physicians seem to take seriously. They often do empirical research with the specific purpose of discovering how many diseases there are, and their method assumes that diseases are natural kinds.

For example, in 1888, Dr Bruce described a condition which he called 'senile rheumatic gout', and which was characterized by muscular pain and morning stiffness. It was later rediscovered and renamed 'polymyalgia rheumatica' by Dr Barber in 1957. It seemed clear that it had a distinct cluster of symptoms:

> Polymyalgia rheumatica is a distinct clinical entity. All the patients described had typical symptoms, a raised erythrocyte sedimentation rate, and no evidence of polymyositis as judged by muscle enzymes, electromyography, and muscle biopsy (Huskisson, Dieppe and Balme, 1977, p.1459).

The main issue that has preoccupied physicians is whether polymyalgia rheumatica is a distinct disease entity. The issue arose because other rheumatic diseases caused muscle pain and stiffness, most importantly the condition of temporal arteritis. This was a condition characterized by a temporal headache, but sometimes preceded by muscle aches and stiffness, and was first described by Dr Huchinson in 1890, and rediscovered later by Drs Horton and Magath in 1932. They wrote: 'The two cases which form the basis of this report probably represent a new clinical syndrome, the etiology of which is still obscure' (Horton and Magath, 1932, p.700). The research into discovering their identity has been concerned, as we would expect, with ascertaining whether the two clusters of symptoms (syndromes) have the same underlying nature. Two researchers write:

> The exact relation between the two syndromes is unknown. Since both are associated with the same histological changes in the arterial wall, they presumably represent different clinical manifestations of a single pathological entity – giant cell arteritis (Harrison and Bevan, 1967, p.640).

This illustrates that physicians do empirical research into the identity and difference among diseases, and shows that they assume that diseases are natural kinds, taking distinct clusters as evidence for distinct natural kinds, but regarding definitive evidence for disease identity as being based upon the identity or difference of the explanatory natures.

The enumeration of psychiatric illnesses also proceeds on the assumption that diseases are natural kinds. For example, psychiatrists have wondered how many depressive illnesses exist. Again, they have looked for a rarity of intermediate forms to support the idea that there are two distinct diseases – reactive and endogenous depression. Robert Kendell writes:

If a psychiatric disorder is to be established as a disease entity on this basis, a natural boundary has therefore to be demonstrated between its symptoms and those of its neighbours. If a putative boundary lies between one syndrome and another this means demonstrating, on an unselected population, that patients with features of both conditions are less common than those with symptoms appropriate to one or the other (Kendell, 1975, p.65).

The belief that disease entities constitute natural kinds is not a recent belief. Thomas Sydenham, the English Hippocrates, wrote in the seventeenth century:

In the first place it is necessary that all diseases be reduced to definite and certain species, and that with the same care which we see exhibited by botanists in their phytologies: since it happens, at present, that many diseases, although included in the same genus, mentioned with the same nomenclature, and resembling one another in several symptoms, are, notwithstanding, different in their natures and require a different medical treatment (Sydenham, 1848, p.13).

This view of the identity of diseases influenced physicians to identify conditions when they believed they had the same nature. One of the most interesting historical examples of this was John Hunter's proof that gonorrhoea and syphilis were the same disease, because they arose from the same poison, that is, had the same nature. This he showed by innoculating himself with pus from a patient with gonorrhoea, but who also (unhappily for Hunter) happened to have syphilis! He wrote:

It has been supposed by many that the gonorrhoea and the chancre arise from two distinct poisons; and their opinion seems to have some foundation, when we consider only the different appearances of the two diseases, and the different methods of cure; which in judging of the nature of many diseases is too often all we have to go by. Yet if we take up this question upon other grounds, and also have recourse to experiments, the result of which we can absolutely depend upon, we shall find this notion erroneous (Hunter, 1786, p.13).

Hunter concluded that syphilis and gonorrhoea were forms of the same disease because they had the same nature in spite of their clinical differences. He thereby illustrated the belief that disease identity consists in identity of the underlying explanatory nature.

As a result of present day empirical research, we have evidence for our belief that disease entities fall into natural kinds. Presently recognized diseases all share a cluster of signs and symptoms – signs and symptoms are not randomly distributed among patients, but cluster instead in certain patients. For example, patients with mumps all share the cluster of fever, malaise, swollen parotid glands, etc. Similarly, patients with gout all share the cluster of painful red joints, tophae, etc. This is good evidence that these patients share different explanatory natures and thereby fall into different natural kinds. And so there is reason to believe that presently recognized disease entities are natural kinds.

In the case of those with mumpy features, we can confirm that they belong to a natural kind because they all share the same nature. But those with gouty features do not share the same explanatory nature, and so do not constitute a single natural kind. Some gouty signs and symptoms are due to the deposition of uric acid in the tissues, while others are due to the deposition of calcium pyrophosphate.

At this point two things could have been concluded about patients with gouty features. Firstly, that they did not constitute a natural kind, and hence that some diseases were not natural kinds. Or secondly, that they did not share the same disease entity, which would mean that diseases are after all natural kinds. What in fact happened was that physicians concluded that those with gouty signs and symptoms did not constitute a disease entity – some had the disease entity of gout, and others had the different disease entity of pseudogout. In fact, whenever a syndrome does not have a single nature, it is concluded that it consists of more than one disease entity.

This seems to show that the question of whether disease entities are natural kinds is not an empirical one – those conditions not constituting a natural kind are simply not treated as a single disease entity. So we know *prior* to our investigations that disease entities will be natural kinds. For example, patients with Bright's disease (patients with proteinuria, dropsy, and morbid changes in the kidney) have turned out not to share an explanatory nature, and because of this the disease is no longer taken to exist.

But if it is not an empirical question whether diseases are natural kinds, it becomes an empirical question just how many presently recognized disease entities actually exist. That is, it becomes an empirical question how many presently recognized disease entities are natural kinds. Are all our present disease categories like Bright's disease?

Skepticism here is not justified. In many cases, we have good evidence that patients with the same disease do have the same explanatory nature. With disease-entities like TB, sickle-cell anaemia, Grave's disease, coeliac disease, and many others, we know what the explanatory natures are, and know that patients with them fall into a natural kind – patients are only taken to have these diseases if they have the appropriate explanatory nature.

However, it turns out that disease entities are not necessarily natural kinds anyway. There are some conditions that physicians classify as diseases (I will call them 'extremal' diseases) but which have natures that are not discontinuous with the normal state. For example, there is no natural boundary between those with essential hypertension and those with normal blood pressure, and hypertensives may have an underlying process that varies only in degree from the norm. The kidneys of hypertensives might just retain more sodium than normal kidneys. As George Pickering remarks in an article entitled 'The nature of hypertension':

> We have grown accustomed to defining a disease, and
> ultimately to ascribing it, to a unique and specific fault with a
> unique and specific cause. The difficulty about the kind of
> essential hypertension that Low and McKeown consider is that
> neither of these steps can be taken. The conviction is steadily
> growing that there is no natural dividing line between normal
> blood pressure and hypertension, and to create one is to create
> an artifact. No specific fault has been found. ... Essential
> hypertension seems to be a disease of a different kind in which
> the fault is not of kind but of degree – the deviation is not
> qualitative but quantitative (Pickering, 1962, p.1298).

If there are indeed conditions that we presently classify as disease entities (for example, essential hypertension) that have underlying processes continuous with the norm, there are three possible positions that we could adopt:

(1) Conditions only differing continuously in degree from the norm are not diseases at all.

(2) Conditions only differing continuously in degree from the norm are diseases, and we are all diseased to a greater or lesser extent!

(3) Conditions only differing continuously in degree from the norm are diseases, and so some diseases are not natural kinds.

Let us explore each of these alternatives in turn.

There are some who advocate the first position: John Patten comments on narcolepsy:

> Narcolepsy is most often seen as an isolated event. The patient is overcome by an irresistible desire to go to sleep, and does so. This may happen while driving a car. It may occur at any time but is exaggerated in circumstances that induce a drowsy state in a normal person such as a stuffy room, a boring lecture, or a heavy meal. In fact, that condition appears to be an exaggeration of normal rather than a disease state (Patten, 1977, p.325).

The argument here seems to be that the condition is not a disease simply because it is an exaggeration of the normal state. In another example, researchers looked for rarity of intermediate forms between Gilbert's disease (raised bilirubin in the blood) and the norm, and reported their findings in an article entitled 'Does Gilbert's disease exist?'

> Both sexes showed skewed distributions for bilirubin con-centration, but analysis of the data showed no evidence of bimodality for either sex. This suggests that people who are now diagnosed as having Gilbert's disease may constitute the upper end of the normal range rather than a disease state (Bailey and Robinson, 1977, p.933).

However, I do not think that this position is viable, because it may turn out that there are simply no diseases at all! It is logically possible that we discover that all the conditions that we have been classifying as diseases merely represent extremes of normal bodily operations. It might look very much like there are discontinuities, but this might be explained by phenomena such as the 'threshold effect'. But it seems absurd to claim that we could discover that there were no human diseases! And so we should reject the first position.

The second position has been included not because there are necessarily any exponents, but because this is one way that one could hang on to the thesis that all diseases are natural kinds. If we wanted to argue that essential hypertension was a natural kind, holding on to the view that all diseases are natural kinds, we would have to say that even normal people had essential hypertension, though of course very much less of it! But this view also seems absurd – it is plainly mistaken to argue that Einstein had very much less of the disease of mental retardation than anybody else!

And this leaves us with the third position – if we want to claim that those with essential hypertension have a disease, and that it is not possible for it to turn out that there are no human diseases, we have to accept that there are some diseases that are not natural kinds. As Robert Kendell puts it:

> [A]n illness may or may not be an entity [= natural kind].
> Whether it is depends on the same criterion as before, whether
> a discontinuity or natural boundary is involved. Down's
> syndrome is an entity because it is caused by, and defined by
> the presence of, a particular chromosomal anomaly which in
> any given individual can only be present or absent. ... Essential
> hypertension is not an entity, in spite of its undoubted genetic
> basis, because that basis is multifactorial, and therefore usually
> present only in partial form (Kendell, 1975, p.68).

Therefore, not all diseases are natural kinds: some have explanatory natures that vary only in degree from the nature of normal individuals.

Does the fact that diseases are not necessarily natural kinds mean that we do not discover the identities and differences that exist among disease-entities? And that we simply invent them to suit our purposes? The answer to these questions is simply 'No'. In spite of the fact that some (perhaps many) disease entities are not natural kinds, disease identity still consists in identity of the explanatory nature. For those diseases that vary only in degree with the norm, this nature has to be quantitatively specified. But this does not mean that we cannot discover that essential hypertension is a distinct disease from diabetes mellitus. If essential hypertensives simply reabsorb more sodium than normal, and diabetics simply have less insulin than normal, we can still discover that these two diseases are distinct by discovering that their natures (even though quantitatively specified) are distinct, and do not vary continuously with one another.

Diseases, then, are not necessarily natural kinds – some diseases may well not constitute a natural kind distinct from the norm. Nevertheless, disease identity consists in identity of the underlying explanatory nature – conditions are not viewed as the same disease entity unless they share the same explanatory nature. This is true also of those diseases that vary continuously with the norm. And because of this, disease identity is something that we discover, rather than invent. We might invent the boundary between disease and the norm (there is no natural boundary between patients with extremal diseases and normal people for us to discover), but we do not invent disease identity.

### Is there a determinate number of pre-existing diseases?

Diseases do not constitute a higher-order natural kind. Because of this, there will not be a determinate number of pre-existing diseases. Whether some condition is or is not a disease depends on what processes we take to be normal, and this is not something that we discover. If we define ageing as normal, it will not be a disease, and we will have $n$ diseases. On the other hand, if we define it as abnormal, we will have $n+1$ diseases. Thus how many diseases there are is not something that is independent of our decisions.

If fish do not constitute a natural kind, the number of fish that there are will be dependent on what we mean by 'fish'. If we mean 'aquatic vertebrate', whales will be counted among fish. If we mean 'aquatic non-mammalian vertebrate', they will not. How many fish there are will depend on what we mean by 'fish'. Since the term 'disease' does not have a NKS either, how many diseases there are will depend on what we mean by 'disease'.

Nevertheless, the weaker thesis that *once disease-status has been settled*, there is a determinate number of diseases existing independently of us, is still defensible. Once we have decided what conditions are normal and what are not, there might be a determinate number of diseases. This is because conditions might fall into lower-order natural kinds. Once the status of ageing has been settled, there might still be a determinate number of disease entities (because there is a determinate number of natural kinds in that domain). However, I will argue that even if all diseases did fall into lower-order natural kinds, it still would not follow that there is a determinate number of them prior to our attempts to count them.

Since I have already shown that not all diseases are natural kinds we can phrase this question differently. It might seem reasonable to infer from the fact that we discover disease-identity, that once we have settled disease-status, we can discover how many individual diseases there are. However, this does not follow. I will argue that the identity of nature is only necessary for the identity of a disease entity, and not sufficient.

Let me start off by asking how many malarial diseases there are. Malaria is an infectious disease caused by four species of Plasmodium – *P. falciparum, P. vivax, P. ovale* and *P. malaria.* Patients with malaria constitute a natural kind. They all share a cluster of general signs and symptoms – patients suffer from paroxysms of rigors and fever, haemolysis and anaemia, etc., and they share a nature that explains these features – they all suffer from parasitization of their red cells by some species of Plasmodium. For example, the rupturing of red cells laden with merozoites and the release of pyrogens explains the paroxysms of fever suffered by the patients.

However each species has its own biology, and is responsible for a different cluster of more specific signs and symptoms. For example, it is because *P. malaria* has an asexual cycle taking 72 hours that patients infected with *P. malaria* have fever and rigors every 72 hours. While it is because *P. ovale* has an asexual cycle taking only 48 hours that fever and rigors occur every 48 hours. Thus on my account of natural kinds, even though patients with malaria constitute a (higher-order) natural kind, patients with each form of malaria also constitute (lower-order) natural kinds.

Lester King raises the question as to how many diseases we have here:

Hippocrates distinguished certain clinical types – the quotidian, the tertian, and the quartan, depending on the periodicity of the paroxysms. The discovery of the specific infectious agent, the plasmodium, opened the door to a clearer understanding, and permitted sharper clinical differentiation. The distinguishable clinical patterns were fairly well correlated with three distinct

183

species of plasmodium. In what we call malaria, how many [disease] entities do we want to distinguish? Should we consider each of the three main clinical types a separate disease entity? (King, 1982, p.154).

Do we have the single disease of malaria, which can take four different but similar forms, or do we have four different but similar diseases, which we might call falciparum malaria, vivax malaria, and so on? The fact that the conditions fall into lower-order and higher-order natural kinds does not help us to count how many disease entities we have here. This is because there is no way of discovering whether a natural kind is a disease-entity natural kind, or what one might call a disease-genus natural kind or a disease-form natural kind. There appears to be nothing about these natural kinds which informs us which is a disease-entity natural kind and which is a disease-genus or disease-form natural kind. How many disease entities we recognize does not depend solely on how many natural kinds there are, for we are still faced with the decision as to *which* natural kinds are to be regarded as disease entities.

Putting this another way, disease identity might consist in the identity of explanatory nature, but this does not enable us to discover how many diseases there are. Patients with malaria all have the same (general) nature – they are all infected by the Plasmodium parasite, but this identity does not enable us to tell whether they thereby belong to the same disease entity or to the same disease genus. We therefore cannot discover how many diseases there are – have to *decide* which natures we take to be the natures of disease entities (rather than the natures of disease genera or forms). The identity of explanatory nature might be *necessary* for disease identity, but it is not *sufficient*. And this means that we cannot discover how many diseases there are – the number also depends on decisions we make about the status of those natures.

This is not a problem confined to malaria. Is insulin-dependent diabetes a distinct disease from insulin-independent diabetes, or simply a different form of the same disease? Does folic acid-deficient megaloblastic anaemia count as a distinct disease or a distinct form from vitamin $B_{12}$-deficient megaloblastic anaemia? Is nutritional rickets a different disease entity from hypophosphatae-mic rickets? Do patients with cerebral beriberi have the same disease as those with wet or dry beriberi? And so on. In each case there are higher- and lower-order natural kinds, and which one is taken to be the disease entity is not something we can discover.

Note that this means that the question 'Does the patient with nutritional rickets have the same disease as the patient with hypo-phosphataemic rickets?' is ambiguous. We can answer it any way we like because the notion of 'same disease' is ambiguous – are we talking about disease forms, entities, or genera? It is much like asking whether English elms are the same trees as American elms – is one talking about the same *species* of tree, or about the same *genus* of tree? What we can say is this – both belong to the broad natural kind of rickets because they share the explanatory nature consisting in defective mineralization of bone. They also fall into distinct lower-order natural kinds because they do not share the more specific way in which this defective mineralization occurs. One has defective mineralization from poor intake of vitamin D, and the other from low levels of phosphate in the blood. There are two correct answers to the question – yes, they both have rickets; no, they do not both have nutritional rickets. The answer to these questions is not something we can *discover*, it is something we have to *decide*. We have to decide what status to ascribe to any natural kind – whether to regard it as a disease entity, or a disease form or genus.

This is not a problem confined to counting diseases either. One might want to know how many substances there are. Different substances fall into natural kinds, and so we might think that we could count the number of substances by counting the natural kinds. But we soon run into difficulties. Does deuterium count as a different substance from hydrogen? They both fall into distinct natural kinds (have different clusters of properties explained by different isotopic natures), but do they belong to different substance natural kinds, or merely substance-form natural kinds? Or does graphite count as a distinct substance from diamond? They both fall into distinct natural kinds (have different clusters of properties explained by different lattice structures of carbon atoms), but do they belong to different substance natural kinds, or merely different substance-form natural kinds? Do we say that hydrogen and deuterium, or graphite and diamond, are merely different forms of the same substance, or do we say that they are different substances altogether?

The reason, I think, why there is not a determinate number of substances (even though they fall into natural kinds), is that substances do not form a higher-order natural kind. And hence we cannot examine the natures of the substances to examine which are and which are not different substances. To make this point clearer, I think that we can argue that there is a determinate number of elements. This is because elements do form a higher-order natural kind – they all share a common type of nature, namely, electronic structure or atomic number. It is this that enables us to say that deuterium is merely a different form of the same element of hydrogen, because it shares with hydrogen its electronic structure, or the number of protons in the nucleus. (It is a different isotopic natural kind because it has a different number of nucleons in its nucleus.) So it is because elements constitute a higher-order natural kind that we can defend the idea that there is a determinate number of them, while conversely it is because substances do not form a higher-order natural kind that there is not.

In a similar way, it is because there is not something about the type of nature that is possessed by disease entities as opposed to disease genera or disease forms, that there is not a determinate number of disease entities. We cannot count the natural kinds with such-and-such a type of nature in order to arrive at a determinate number of disease entities, for they lack a specific type of nature different from disease genera or disease forms.

In biology, one can count the number of species (as opposed to species forms or genera) by counting the number of natures that maintain reproductive isolation. In this way, even though we might argue that one race of dog or man or bird is a distinct natural kind from another (they have different clusters of characteristics explained by different genetic natures), they are not different *species* because their natures do not have the crucial feature of ensuring reproductive isolation, and it is this feature of an organism's nature that makes it a distinct species (as opposed to a distinct race or genus).

If being a natural kind is not sufficient for a condition to be a disease entity – if identity of nature is not sufficient for disease identity, it is natural to ask what else is needed. Some might argue that the different forms of malaria are all forms of the same disease because they have very similar explanatory natures. However, this suggestion is not very helpful. For we might with equal plausibility (or rather, implausibility) argue that there is just one viral infectious disease – all these are characterized by a very similar explanatory nature: in all cases, a virus enters the body, attaches itself to the cells of the body, injects its nuclear material, hijacks the cell's metabolic machinery to reproduce more of itself, with the consequent rupture of the cell to release the viral products. But this similarity does not tempt us to conclude that we only have a single disease, 'viritis'.

So we cannot use the notion of 'sufficient similarity' of the nature to determine which natural kind counts as a disease entity natural kind. Caroline Whitbeck suggests that it is the therapeutic usefulness of the classification that determines which natural kind is a disease entity natural kind:

> What is distinctive about disease entities as opposed to other natural kinds, such as chemical compounds or biologic species, is the conspicuousness of the clinical goals of prevention and treatment in the choice of criteria that are used to define disease entities and to discriminate among them. . . . The aim [of disease classification] is not the precise identification of a fully defined clinical entity, but whatever degree of identification is necessary to achieve the best outcome for the patient and to prevent the spread of disease. Far from being the central activity of medicine, the identification of disease entities derives what importance it has from its role in informing therapy and prevention (Whitbeck, 1981, p.321).

Perhaps it is the identity of treatment plus the identity of nature that is sufficient for disease identity. Perhaps the forms of malaria are taken to be forms of the same disease because they share the same nature *and* they can be treated in the same way.

However, I think this move is mistaken. Firstly, it is not true that all forms of malaria can be treated in the same way. We might be able to *prevent* them in the same way by preventing bites from *Anopheline* mosquitos, but there are many strains of *P. falciparum* that are chloroquine resistant, and so cannot be treated in the same way that the non-resistant forms can. But we do not conclude that these forms constitute a distinct disease entity.

Secondly, there are many distinct diseases that at some level share the same nature, and which can also be treated in the same way. For example, many diseases such as syphilis, impetigo, pneumococcal pneumonia, etc., share the nature of being infections by penicillin-sensitive organisms, and can (therefore) be treated in the same way by penicillin, but this does not ensure that syphilis is the same disease as impetigo. In addition, if all viral infections or

187

cancers could be treated in the same way, this would not ensure that there was only one viral disease ('viritis') and only one cancerous disease.

I am not able to give necessary and sufficient conditions for disease identity because I do not think there are any. All we can say is that some natural kinds are accorded the status of being disease entities, and others accorded the status of being disease forms or genera. I suspect that what natural kinds we regard as disease entity natural kinds is in part due to historical accident. It is because malaria was considered to be a single disease entity that we regard it in this way now. However, this cannot be the whole story because gout too was regarded as a single disease entity, but we recognize now that there are many different disease entities that produce gouty symptoms. Nevertheless, having the same explanatory nature is *necessary* for being the same disease entity.

In summary, diseases are not necessarily natural kinds – there are diseases that have no natural boundary with normality. Nevertheless disease (whether disease entity, genus or form) identity still consists in the identity of explanatory nature. But I have shown that this does not mean that there is a determinate number of diseases existing prior to our taxonomies. What counts as a disease entity natural kind is a matter of *decision*, and not discovery.

Disease (whether disease entity, genus, or form) identity is still something that we can discover. This is because identity of explanatory nature is necessary and sufficient for *some order* of disease identity. However, we cannot argue that we can discover disease entity identity. This is because even though identity of nature is necessary for disease entity identity, it is not sufficient. If we discover that the natures differ, we cannot conclude that the disease entities are different – they might be natures of different disease *forms* and not disease *entities*. Similarly, if we discover that the natures are the same, we cannot conclude that the disease-entities are the same – they might be the natures of the same disease *genus* but not the same disease *entity*.

Thus there is only a grain of truth in TR as applied to the classification of diseases. Although we cannot defend the idea that disease status is discovered and not invented, we *can* argue that some order of disease identity is discovered. We cannot argue that we can discover disease-entity identity (or disease-genus identity), because we have to *decide* which natures are the natures of disease entities, and which are the natures of disease genera. There is no fact that reflects what sort of nature with which we are dealing. But there is some fact that enables us to discover some order of disease identity or difference. If we can defend the idea that disease terms purport to pick out such natures, we could argue that there is at least a part of nosology that can be true or false, correct or mistaken. I will examine the semantics of disease terms in Chapter 11.

# CHAPTER 11
# THE SEMANTICS OF DISEASE TERMS

## Introduction

In this chapter I will examine the semantics of disease terms. This is with a view to assessing whether TR, the thesis that classificatory systems can be correct or incorrect, is true of nosology. In order for TR to be true of some domain, we have seen that two conditions have to obtain. Firstly, the objects classified in that domain must fall into natural kinds. If they do not, then there will be nothing for the taxonomy to reflect. And secondly, the terms used to classify those objects must purport to pick out natural kinds. If they do not, then we cannot convict the taxonomy of error.

In order, then, for there to be some content to the claim that our nosologies can be mistaken, disease terms must have some form of NKS. In the last chapter I argued that disease identity (whether identity of disease entity, genus, or form) consisted in the identity of explanatory nature. This is true even for those diseases that are not natural kinds. If the claim that we *discover* disease identity is to be made good, the thesis that disease terms refer to the explanatory natures or real essences must be defended. If disease terms express nominal essences, then disease identity can be invented by choosing one nominal essence for any disease term rather than another.

In Chapter 2 I defended a Combined Theory for the semantics of terms that purported to pick out natural kinds. On this theory, the terms have a descriptive sense, but one that is not sufficient to fix the reference or extension of that term. This is fixed by the actual nature of the objects causally related (in the right sort of way) to the use of the term. I argued that this descriptive sense was necessary to disambiguate the reference of classificatory terms. It is ambiguous to say that anything with the same nature as *that* is an elm – is one referring to its species nature or genus nature? It is only if terms have a certain descriptive sense that we can disambiguate this reference. I also argued that it is an empirical question just what semantics our terms have. Studying the use of such terms, there is considerable evidence that they have a Combined theory meaning.

## What medical language do we speak?

There is considerable evidence that our disease terms have a NKS. I have argued that evidence must not come from our (sometimes conflicting) linguistic intuitions. It must come instead from the actual usage of disease terms. The most striking support comes from the use of disease terms in existential denials and identity statements.

If disease terms purport to pick out natural kinds, and they fail to do so, we expect physicians to conclude that such diseases do not exist. And this is exactly what we find. For example, Richard Bright described a condition that presented with proteinuria, dropsy, and morbid changes in the kidney. However, it was soon realized that the conditions falling into the category of 'Bright's disease' did not constitute a natural kind (of any order). Physicians concluded that Bright's disease did not exist, which is what we would expect them to say if the term had a NKS.

Similarly, in the nineteenth century the disease of floating kidney or nephroptosis was well recognized. This 'disease' could produce a variety of symptoms, including abdominal pain, tenderness over the kidneys, nausea, vomiting, dysuria, haematuria, etc. It was supposed to be due to a kidney that was not tethered properly. However, in this century it was realized that such a group of patients did not constitute a natural kind (of any order). As a result, physicians concluded that nephroptosis does not exist (Murphy, 1972, p. 209).

If our disease terms have a NKS, then we expect conditions to be identified if they are found to have the same explanatory nature, and conditions to be differentiated if they do not. And this is precisely what we do find. In the late nineteenth century, the Russian psychiatrist Korsakoff described the psychotic condition characterized by severe long-term memory loss, which now bears his name – Korsakoff's psychosis. The German physician Wernicke described a different clinical condition characterized by delirium, which we now call Wernicke's encephalopathy. However, pathological investigation showed that these patients suffered from the same neurological damage. Later, the discovery was made that they were both due to the deficiency of thiamine. Thiamine deficiency also results in peripheral neuropathy and cardiac failure, conditions that had been classified under the disease of beriberi. As a result of these discoveries, physicians concluded that all these clinical pictures were forms of the same disease of beriberi. Patients with beriberi can have peripheral neuropathy (dry beriberi), cardiac failure (wet beriberi), or delirium and psychosis (cerebral beriberi). It was concluded that they were after all the same disease (because they had the same explanatory nature) (Victor, Adams and Collins, 1971).

Similarly, when general paresis of the insane was first recognized, it was not realized that it was a form of syphilis. However, the first clue that it was came from Fournier, who in 1875 found that 65 per cent of general paretics had a history of syphilis, while only 10 per cent of other mentally ill patients had suffered from syphilis in the past. Finally, Noguchi and Moore in 1913 demonstrated treponema pallidum in the brain of syphilitics. It was because general paresis of the insane had the same nature as primary (and secondary) syphilis that it was concluded that it was a form of syphilis (Henry, 1941).

Conversely, patients with haemophilia are not the only patients that can present with the identical clinical picture of bruising and bleeding. Some patients with such a clinical pattern do not suffer from the deficiency of clotting factor 8 that is responsible for haemophilia, but instead have a deficiency of factor 9. As a result, these patients have been viewed as having the different disease entity called 'Christmas disease'. It is because terms purport to pick out natural kinds that such conclusions are drawn.

So it seems to be the case that disease terms have a NKS. If this is so, and if (as we have argued is the case) diseases fall into natural kinds, then TR will be true of the classification of diseases (at the level of disease entities). That is, certain classifications will be mistaken because they identify disease entities that do not share the same nature, while others will be correct because they differentiate disease entities with different natures.

This will explain why it is that physicians take there to be a factual issue at stake over whether certain diseases are identical or different. For example, we have seen that physicians comment on the issue of whether Werdnig–Hoffman's disease is the same as Kugelberg–Welander in such terms: 'It is not known at present whether each of these disorders is a separate disease entity' and 'It is questionable whether they represent distinct entities'. We have seen physicians comment on the issue of whether polymyalgia rheumatica is the same disease as temporal arteritis in such terms: 'The exact relation between the two syndromes is unknown' and 'The question posed by the condition is one of identity'. They would not speak in this way unless they believed that there was a factual issue at stake.

In addition, they talk as if the question of identity is settled by the discovery of the identity of the underlying natures. Some physicians comment on the relation between polymyalgia rheumatica and temporal arteritis:

> The histological findings in our material strongly support the view that polymyalgia rheumatica and temporal arteritis are different manifestations of one and the same pathological process, the underlying cause being an arteritis (Hamrin, Jonsson and Landberg, 1964, p. 397).

Here it is assumed that there is a fact of the matter about the relation of the two conditions, and that this fact involves the identity or difference of the underlying natures.

However, it might seem premature to conclude that disease terms have a NKS. It might be argued that disease terms do not have a NKS because we might have to conclude that there are no diseases if it turns out that there are no such natural kinds. Let me illustrate this argument with a parallel one for trees:

(1) Trees might not share a real essence.
(2) If trees do not share a real essence, and 'tree' purports to refer to a real essence, we would have to conclude that trees do not exist.
(3) It is not possible that trees do not exist.
(4) Therefore, 'tree' does not purport to refer to a natural kind.

It might be felt that this argument is not valid, because it *is* possible that trees do not exist – for example, we might discover that they are holograms projected by malicious Martians. But we can modify the argument thus:

(1) Given that what we believe of trees so far – namely, that they are plants, etc. – is true, it is possible that they do not share a real essence.

(2) If trees do not share a real essence, and 'tree' purports to refer to a real essence, we would have to conclude that trees do not exist.

(3) Given that what we believe of trees so far is true, it is not possible that they do not exist.

(4) Therefore, 'tree' does not purport to refer to a natural kind.

So the argument, in essence, is that some terms do not have a NKS because we would not conclude that such a kind does not exist (if we were to discover that no real essence was shared). And the claim is that we would not conclude that particular diseases do not exist if we discovered they do not share a real essence.

However, I have just shown that this is precisely what we *do* conclude. We conclude that Bright's disease and nephroptosis do not exist precisely because they do not constitute natural kinds. And therefore this argument fails.

There is another objection that might be levelled at the view that disease terms have a NKS. It will be objected that if disease terms purport to pick out natural kinds, then we will have to conclude that extremal diseases do not exist when we discover that they do not constitute natural kinds. If essential hypertensives simply reabsorb more sodium from their kidneys than normal, and there is no natural boundary between them and normotensives, they will not constitute a natural kind. But then we will have to conclude that essential hypertension does not exist! And this seems to show that disease terms do not have a NKS because we would not conclude that essential hypertension does not exist.

There are a number of positions that could be adopted here:

(1) We could conclude that essential hypertension does not exist, and hope that most diseases will be natural kinds so that we will not be forced to say that there are no diseases!

(2) We could conclude that disease terms do not have a NKS.

(3) We could conclude that disease terms have a NKS, but that any class of objects that shares an explanatory nature (even if this only varies continuously with the natures of other kinds) constitutes a natural kind.

(4) We could conclude that disease terms initially have a NKS, but that when it is discovered that they do not pick out natural kinds, their meaning could *change* to assume a DS, thereby

enabling us to preserve the truth of sentences containing those terms.

(5) We could conclude that disease terms have a NKS, but that all that is necessary for such terms to successfully refer is for the class of objects to share an explanatory nature (even of a quantitatively defined variety), whether or not they constitute a natural kind.

I will look at each position in turn.

The first position is unpalatable – it would be absurd to commit ourselves to the possibility that there are no diseases. Since it *is* possible that all diseases have natures that only vary in degree from the normal population, and since we would not say that there were no diseases, the first position is unacceptable.

Concluding that disease terms do not have a NKS would fly in the face of all the evidence that they do indeed purport to refer to real essences. The use of disease terms especially in negative existential and identity claims provides strong support for the theory that disease terms have a NKS. Thus the second position is also incorrect.

I have argued that we should accept an account of natural kinds in terms of which there must be 'natural divisions' among classes that constitute different natural kinds. It is because different cloud genera do not have natural divisions among their natures that they do not constitute natural kinds. I have argued for this view of natural kinds because one of the central ideas behind the concept of natural kinds is the idea that they exist independently of us and can be discovered. But if there are no natural divisions between the classes, we cannot be said to *discover* that there are distinct kinds of things. Therefore, the idea of a natural kind incorporates the idea that there are discontinuities (which we can discover) among natural kinds. And so the third position is also wrong.

The fourth position is not correct either. The discovery that 'Bright's disease' does not pick out a natural kind did not lead to the term assuming a descriptive meaning and expressing the nominal essence of 'syndrome of proteinuria, dropsy, and morbid changes in the kidney'. We do not say that Bright's disease exists after all.

It is the last position that is correct in spite of the seemingly paradoxical implication that terms with a NKS can successfully refer even if the objects picked out do not fall into a natural kind. This position has two virtues. Firstly, it avoids the problems of the other positions. Secondly, it explains why terms like 'essential hypertension' behave as if they had a NKS. Suppose we discovered that essential hypertension was due to the excessive renal reabsorption of sodium. No one would be taken to have essential hypertension unless they had a condition with this nature. And this shows that the term has a NKS.

In addition, if it turned out that there were two different natures underlying essential hypertension, and that they did not share any more general nature, we would conclude that there were two disease entities mistaken as a single disease entity. Again, this supports the view that even terms referring to extremal disease have a NKS.

However, there is one problem with this view. It might be argued that normal people have the same process that underlies essential hypertension (although to a lesser degree), and therefore we should conclude that we all have essential hypertension. That is, if we define 'essential hypertensives' in terms of whoever has the same on-going process as *these people*, we would have to conclude that we are all suffering from essential hypertension.

But this does not follow. Just as the reference of terms like 'water', 'hydrogen', 'elm', and so on, is disambiguated by a minimal description, so the term 'essential hypertension' can be shown not to refer to normal people. For example, when we wish to refer to the species of elm, the description of the kind as a 'species' disambiguates the reference (from the genus).

Similarly, it is the description of the kind of hypertensives as having a disease that disambiguates the reference (from normal people). Since it is only hypertensives that have renal reabsorption of sodium to the degree that is harmful – part of the meaning of being a disease – it is only this degree that constitutes the real essence of essential hypertension. And hence normal people do not have it.

If disease terms have a NKS, is their extension determined by the Causal theory or by the Combined theory? There is a theoretical argument that favours the combined theory over the Causal theory, If we spoke causalese, our terms would be too ambiguous. The extension of a term is fixed by whatever has the same nature as some sample object. However, there is no such thing as *the* nature. The nature of any disease could be taken to be the *cause* rather than the *process*.

And so it would not be clear whether impetigo is a form of the same disease as puerperal fever because they are both caused by streptococcus, or whether glandular fever is the same disease as Burkitt's lymphoma because they are both caused by the Epstein Barr virus. Conversely, it would not be clear whether squamus carcinoma of the skin caused by irradiation was the same disease as squamus carcinoma of the skin caused by arsenic.

Hilary Putnam believes that the cause of a disease is its nature:

> What we should like to say is this: there is (we presume) in the world something – say, a virus – which normally causes such-and-such symptoms. Perhaps other diseases occasionally (rarely) produce these same symptoms in a few patients. When a patient has these symptoms we say he has 'multiple sclerosis' – but, of course, we are prepared to say that we were mistaken if the etiology turns out to be abnormal. And we are prepared to classify sicknesses as cases of multiple sclerosis, even if the symptoms are rather deviant, if it turns out that the *underlying condition* was the virus that causes multiple sclerosis, and the deviancy was, say, random variation (Putnam, 1976b, p. 310).

Putnam correctly points out that disease terms have a NKS, but is mistaken in thinking that the nature of a disease is its cause. As William Goosens argues:

> Putnam's reason for his claim is that all along the cause, known or unknown, is our conception of the disease, so that the symptoms never formed our conception. While I agree that the symptoms never formed our conception, it is not correct that cause is the general semantical category for disease (Goosens, 1977, p. 135).

Goosens argues for this by asking whether someone who developed a tuberculous inflammatory reaction in response to some new insecticide would have TB. He argues that they both have TB in spite of the difference in cause. I have cautioned against using linguistic intuitions to support such arguments, and prefer to rely on the fact that our actual judgments of disease identity and difference are simply not based on identity or difference of cause.

If different causes produce the same process, they cause the same disease. It is because irradiation and arsenic cause the same process that they cause the same disease. On the other hand, if the same cause results in different processes, it causes a number of different diseases. It is because the process underlying impetigo is different from that underlying puerperal fever that these streptococcal diseases are distinct. This means that the 'semantical category', as Goosens puts it, for disease entities is not cause, but process. It is because 'disease' has the descriptive meaning of picking out processes that we do not treat *mere* differences or identities in cause as sufficient for differences or identities of disease.

To take Putnam's example, multiple sclerosis may well be caused by the measles virus, but we would not conclude that multiple sclerosis is the same disease as measles! This is because the terms 'measles' and 'multiple sclerosis' do not refer to just any nature – they refer to the explanatory *process* rather than the *cause*. Thus they do not refer to the virus, and having the same cause will not mean that they are the same disease. On the other hand, if we were to discover that the same process going on in patients with Parkinson's disease is also responsible for Alzheimer's disease, we *will* conclude that they are forms of the same disease.

Thus the fact that we do not take mere identity or difference of cause as sufficient for identity or difference of disease, and the fact that we require there to be identity or difference in the underlying process for there to be identity or difference of disease, shows that disease terms have a descriptive sense that excludes causes from being candidates of the nature of diseases. Diseases are processes, and because the term has this much descriptive sense, our reference is not radically ambiguous. This supports the Combined theory over the Causal theory.

Thus it seems that we have evidence that our disease terms have a NKS. In addition, it seems that the use of our terms conform to the predictions of the Combined theory. The minimal sense of any disease term consists in the idea that such a condition is both a process and harmful.

## A taxonomy of terms

Disease terms are not the only terms that occur in medical discourse. There are also terms that refer to signs and symptoms, for example 'pallor' or 'weakness'. Then there are terms that refer to syndromes (constellations of signs and symptoms), for example 'Acquired Immune Deficiency Syndrome' or 'dementia'. And finally there are terms that describe the nature of diseases, for

example 'hypothyroidism' or 'mitral stenosis'. Not all of them may
have a NKS. John Mackie argues that there are two sorts of disease
or ailment terms:

> The names of diseases and ailments also seem to fall into two
> classes: 'malaria' is annexed to its real essence, and probably
> was so annexed even before its real essence (the precise nature
> of the infection, the malarial parasite) was known, but
> 'jaundice' is annexed to a group of symptoms. 'Measles' and
> 'schizophrenia' are like 'malaria': though these illnesses are
> identified by sets of symptoms which pick out paradigm cases,
> these names are intended to refer not to the set of symptoms
> but to whatever underlying physical or mental condition
> commonly produces those symptoms: this same conditon
> would still be measles (or schizophrenia) even if for some
> reason it failed, in a particular patient, to produce the usual
> symptoms. Is it important that there are a measles virus and a
> malarial parasite, that is, that though these diseases are not
> substances, each is related to a sort of substance? I think not:
> there is no schizophrenia microbe. What such examples show is
> that it is not the difference between substances and non-
> substances that matters here, in the sense of the distinction
> between items which are supposed to 'subsist by themselves'
> and items which are not, but rather the difference between
> cases where it is useful or fruitful to think and speak pre-
> ferentially of a possibly unknown or inadequately known
> 'nature' and cases where it is more appropriate to concentrate
> attention on a *syndrome*, a collection of symptoms or
> superficially observable features (Mackie, 1976, p.99).

Mackie makes three claims here. First, that disease terms have a
NKS – they purport to pick out natural kinds by referring to the
explanatory natures of those conditions. Second, that such terms
have always had such a semantics. Third, that there is another class
of terms which purport to pick out symptoms or syndromes – that
is, have a DS, and which do not purport to pick out natural kinds.

I will start with the last claim first. There are three important
classes in terms that have a DS. Firstly, many terms that describe
certain signs and symptoms, for example, 'pallor' and 'weakness',
have a descriptive meaning. If they did not, we could never gather

together objects into likely natural kinds in virtue of their satisfying a cluster of descriptive predicates.

Secondly, terms that describe the real essence also have a DS. If they did not, we could never tell when objects sharing a cluster of properties belonged to the same natural kind. It is in virtue of their satisfying the same description of their natures that they belong to the same natural kind. 'Gold' has a NKS, because nothing is gold unless it has whatever nature is shared by those objects standing in the right sort of causal relation to the use of the term. But we confirm that substances are gold if their natures satisfy the description 'atomic number 79', assuming this is the nature of gold. This phrase has a DS, because nothing has this property unless it has 79 protons in its nucleus. Similarly, 'Grave's disease' has a NKS because nobody has the disease unless they have whatever nature is shared by those who stand in the right sort of causal relation to the use of that term. But 'hypothyroidism' has a DS because no one has this disease unless their thyroids are hypofunctioning.

Finally, there are many terms that refer to constellations of signs and symptoms without relation to underlying processes. For example, the term 'dementia' refers to a group of acquired and irreversible cognitive defects, and does not imply that the patient has any one disease (for example, Alzheimer's disease) rather than another (for example, multi-infarct dementia). Whoever satisfies the description encapsulated in the term 'dementia', has dementia – the term has a DS.

Although some terms referring to signs and symptoms have a DS, 'jaundice' does not. It does not refer just to the signs and symptoms that occur with liver disease, namely the yellowing of the skin and sclera. The term refers to the underlying pathological state that *explains* these signs and symptoms – the raised bilirubin level in the blood. Someone with the same signs and symptoms, but who does not have the same nature (of raised bilirubin) is not jaundiced. For example, the ingestion of excessive quantities of vitamin A can lead to carotinaemia, and this also produces a yellowing of the skin and sclera. But this is not jaundice. So while Mackie might be right to think that *some* terms (like 'yellowing of the skin') have a descriptive sense, he draws the line in the wrong place – there are many more terms that have a NKS than there are disease entity terms.

Many physicians might support Mackie in claiming that terms that ostensibly refer to syndromes (and not disease entities) also have a NES. Such terms might include 'Cushing's syndrome', 'diabetes mellitus', 'anaemia', and so on.

> Diabetes Mellitus should be viewed as a description rather than a diagnosis [of a specific disease entity]. It describes a class of disease characterized by chronically elevated blood sugar concentration often accompanied by other clinical and biochemical abnormalities. ... As a term, 'diabetes mellitus' is comparable to 'anaemia' or 'hypertension'. It draws attention to a major identifying characteristic and indicates a set of therapeutic options, predictable complications, and possible causes. In recent years, a variety of causative mechanisms has been more clearly defined. Diabetes Mellitus is thus most usefully regarded as a synonym for persisting hyperglycaemia and not the title of a single disease entity (Keen, 1981, p.327).

While it is the case that the term 'diabetes' is like the terms 'anaemia' and 'hypertension', it does not follow from this that the term has a descriptive meaning. Patients who present with the syndrome of palpitations, shortness of breath, fatigue, pallor, dizziness, etc., are often suffering from one form of anaemia. Anaemic patients constitute a natural kind – they all share a cluster of signs and symptoms, and have a common underlying nature to explain this cluster – a low haemaglobin concentration. Because someone only has anaemia if they have this same explanatory nature, 'anaemia' refers to the real essence of the condition, and is not synonymous with the description of the resulting syndrome. A number of other conditions can present with the same clinical picture, for example cardiac failure, but the patients would not have anaemia because they would not have the same nature as those with pernicious anaemia, etc. 'Anaemia', then, does not mean 'syndrome with palpitations, pallor, etc'. It might be that there are a number of different disease entities of anaemia, and this is why one speaks of the anaemias (plural), but this does not mean that the term must be a descriptive one, and cannot refer to the real essence of the condition and pick out a higher-order natural kind.

Similarly, it does not follow from the fact that the class of diabetic patients does not constitute a disease entity natural kind, that the term 'diabetes' has a descriptive meaning. The important thing is that diabetics constitute a natural kind (albeit a higher-order one), and that we do not take those who present with a similar clinical picture to have diabetes unless they also have the same nature as those who fall into the natural kind of diabetics – namely, impaired insulin functioning. And so it would seem that the term 'diabetes' functions like any other natural kind term – it might not pick out a disease entity, but that is beside the point. Thus the class of medical terms that have a DS is narrower than some suspect.

I have already argued for Mackie's first claim. Disease terms are not synonymous with descriptions of syndromes. Thus we accept that different diseases can result in the same clinical syndrome, and conversely that the same disease can result in different clinical syndromes. Christmas disease and haemophilia can result in the same clinical picture, while polio can present as a 'flu-like illness, meningitis, and classical flaccid paralysis. If the terms were synonymous with a description of the syndromes, identity statements would have different truth values from the ones that they actually possess.

The second claim that disease terms have always purported to refer to real essences requires a much more detailed historical argument than I have space for here. It might be instructive, nevertheless, to look at the evolution of some disease terms in order to assess this claim. I will show that disease terms have not always had the same meaning.

The term 'fibrositis' was introduced by Sir William Gowers in 1904 to refer to patients who were suffering from muscle pains, stiffness, and localized tenderness (Gowers, 1904). Such cases of 'rheumatism' had been known since antiquity, but what was new was Gowers' idea that the condition was due to inflammation of fibrous tissue, hence the suffix 'itis' taken to imply inflammation. At this stage it is clear that the term not only purported to pick out a real essence, but also to *characterize* that essence as satisfying a certain description, namely, that of being an inflammation of fibrous tissue. Had Gowers discovered that most of these patients did not have this nature of fibrous inflammation, and that a minority did, he would undoubtedly have regarded only the latter as having fibrositis. Having that particular sort of nature was essential for being a case of fibrositis – the term had a DS.

For a time the disease of fibrositis was accepted, and received some support from the pathological studies of Ralph Stockman who believed he had demonstrated that these patients were indeed suffering from inflammatory changes in their fibrous tissue, which he called 'fibrositic nodules' (Stockman, 1904). However sub-sequent studies failed to reveal any inflammatory changes in fibrous tissue – many of these patients were found to be suffering from other diseases, like giant cell arteritis. As a result, physicians began to claim that there was no such inflammatory disease as fibrositis. The term still had its descriptive meaning.

Recently workers have isolated a group of patients with the fibrositic-like clinical picture who are not suffering from other disease like giant cell arteritis. A new explanatory nature has been postulated:

> The essential feature of 'fibrositis' is exaggerated tenderness at widely distributed but specifically located sites. .... Assuming that 'fibrositis' is a disorder of pain modulation, it is tempting to speculate that the fundamental abnormality is an absolute or relative endorphine deficiency (Smythe, 1979, p.830).

What is interesting is that the term 'fibrositis' is used in quotation, indicating that the term possessed a descriptive meaning (implying inflammation of fibrous tissue) which it no longer carries. If the term did not have a descriptive meaning, there would be no need to indicate that one was not using the work to imply fibrous inflammation, and hence no need to use the quotations.

It now looks like the term 'fibrositis' has a NKS. If it turns out that such patients are not suffering from endorphine deficiency, but have some other nature, they will still be suffering from fibrositis (so long as they have *some* explanatory nature in common). Thus we have a term that started out with a DS and came to acquire a NKS. What is also significant about this example is that it shows that there are some disease terms that not only purport to pick out real essences, but also to characterize them, and hence have a DS.

Similarly, the term 'hysteria' originally purported to pick out a class of female patients who were not only taken to share a real essence explaining a diversity of symptoms from abdominal pain to feelings of suffocation ('globus hystericus'), but also taken to have a nature that satisfied a certain description. All the patients were supposed to be suffering from the ill effects of a migratory uterus, hence the term 'hysteria' which is derived from the Greek word for womb. A woman suffering from suffocating feelings not taken to be due to a migratory uterus was not classified as having hysteria. Instead, she might be seen as suffering from asthma (panting)

203

(Veith, 1965a). Similarly, patients who clinically resembled epileptics but who were suffering from migratory uteri were classified as suffering from hysteria and not epilepsy. Hence the term started out with a DS.

Today, the term is still in use, but we have long since recognized that the uterus is not able to migrate and cause such symptoms, and that such patients must be suffering from some other underlying condition. Whoever has the same nature as such patients is taken to have hysteria, and hence the term 'hysteria' has now assumed a NKS.

Similarly, 'melancholia' was a term used by physicians long after the Hippocratic theory of humours was rejected. But the term used to imply an excess of black bile, hence the name 'melan-cholia' meaning black bile (Lewis, 1934, p.1459). And so its sense here must have changed from a DS to a NKS such that it no longer carried the implication that the nature of the condition consisted in the excess of black bile. Another example is the term 'tumour', which was a term that literally meant (in ancient Greek) 'swelling'. Tumours included both abscesses, oedema, as well as cancer. For example, Galen classified tumours into (1) *supra naturum* (exceeding nature) such as the callous formation uniting a fracture; (2) *secundam naturam* (according to nature) such as the gravid uterus; and (3) *praeter naturum* (contrary to nature) a larger group including cancer, oedema, and abscesses (Kardinal and Yarbro, 1979, p.398). Only later did the term assume a NKS such that only something with the same nature as any neoplasm counted as a tumour.

It is worth noting that even though these terms had a DS, the physicians of the past still viewed the conditions as natural kinds. Any symptom that was due to a migrating uterus, that is, had the nature of hysteria, was hysteria. And unless a symptom was due to a migrating uterus, it was not hysteria. Similarly, it was because excess black bile was thought to lead to abdominal pain, that this too was considered to be a feature of melancholia (Jobe, 1976, pp.217–31).

Let us look at the term 'myxoedema'. In 1873 Sir William Gull read before the Clinical Society a paper entitled 'A cretinoid state supervening in adult life in women':

> That the state is a substantive and definite one, no one will
> doubt who has had fair opportunity of observing it. And that it

is allied to the cretin state would appear from the formative features, the changes in the lips and tongue, the character of the hands, the alterations and conditions of locomotion, the peculiarities, though slight, of the mental state (Gull, 1873, p.180).

It is clear that he was referring to women suffering from hypo-thyroidism, and took himself to be describing a disease entity.

Dr William Ord first introduced the term 'myxoedema' in 1878 to refer to such a condition after he had examined the pathology of such patients:

As regards the class of cases immediately in question, my suggestion is that the whole collection of symptoms are related as effects to the jelly-like swelling of the connective tissue, chiefly if not entirely consisting in an overgrowth of the mucus-yielding element. ... Accordingly, I propose to give the name myxoedema to the affection. ... [T]he name is only intended to represent the condition, and does not profess to involve an explanation of its causes (Ord, 1978, p.57).

It might be suspected that the term 'myxoedema' had a DS describing the pathological lesion. But in 1888, a Committee of the Clinical Society of London reported on the status of myxoedema as a new disease. Some of their conclusions were:

That myxoedema is a well defined disease.... That clinical and pathological observations, respectively, indicate in a decisive way, that the one condition common to all cases is destructive change of the thyroid gland (Committee's Report 1888).

Thus it appears that only a few years after Sir William Ord had proposed that the 'essential lesion' was the mucoid edema, the term 'myxoedema' was being used to refer to a condition which physicians believed was a disorder of the thyroid gland. If the term 'myxoedema' did have a DS, they ought to have concluded that they were mistaken to think that such patients had that disease. As Hun and Prudden reported in the *American Journal of Medical Science* in 1888: 'However obscure the function of the thyroid gland may be, there can be little doubt that its lesion is the essential lesion of myxoedema' (Hun and Prudden, 1888, p.140). It seems that the most plausible hypothesis to account for this continued use of the term, in spite of the change of belief as to what the essential lesion consisted in, is that the term had a NKS and not a descriptive meaning. Later, physicians were to separate out a number of distinct disease entities of the thyroid that could result in such a clinical picture. As a result of these discoveries, the term 'myxoedema' is no longer taken to refer to a disease entity, but instead a whole class of disease entities that result in hypo-thyroidism.

Thus it appears from this small sample of the history of disease terms that they were not always used to pick out whatever happened to be the explanatory nature of the condition standing in the right causal relation to the use of the term. Sometimes terms were introduced with a descriptive meaning. So even though our disease terms now have a NKS of the Combined Theory variety, they need not always have had such a meaning.

In conclusion, then, most disease terms have a NKS. This is true even if they pick out patients that do not constitute a natural kind, as do essential hypertensives. There are other terms describing signs and symptoms, like 'pallor', those describing syndromes, like 'dementia', and those describing the nature of certain diseases and pathological conditions, like 'hypothyroidism', that have a DS. Some terms referring to signs and syndromes, like 'jaundice' and 'diabetes mellitus', in spite of appearances to the contrary, also have a NKS. Finally, I have argued that disease terms can change their meaning – such as 'hysteria', 'melancholy', and 'fibrositis'. They start out with a DS, and later assume a NKS. Thus they have not always had a NKS.

Because most of our disease terms have a NKS, there is a grain of TR in nosology. The grain consists in the fact that we do not invent disease identity (at any level), but rather we discover it. We discover it because most disease terms purport to pick out conditions sharing the same nature, and because we can discover whether conditions do in fact share the same nature. Even if conditions do not fall into lower-level natural kinds, we can discover disease identity because this consists in identity of nature, and this is something that we can discover. So there can be parts of any nosology that are correct (when the terms purporting to pick out natural kinds succeed in doing so), or incorrect (when the terms purporting to pick out natural kinds fail to do so). Of course we have seen that TR is not true of the whole of the nosology. Diseases and pathological conditions do not constitute natural kinds and the terms 'disease' and 'pathological condition' do not purport to pick out such kinds.

## CONCLUSION
# WHEN IS A DISEASE NOT A DISEASE?

**Non-existent diseases**

By way of a summary, let us see just when a putative disease fails to earn its disease status. Many candidates for disease status have been proposed through the ages and some have not held on to their claim to be the diseases. It is worth examining why.

Some putative diseases are not diseases because they do not cause the individual any harm. Axillary odour, which is uncommon among Japanese, but usual among Caucasians, was taken by the Japanese to be a disease which they called 'osmidrosis axillae', and one that warranted hospitalization and exemption from the army. Such a condition is not a disease because the condition does not do the individual any harm – osmidrosis axillae does not exist (Wing, 1978, pp.16–7).

This example is complicated by the fact that the Japanese find axillary odour offensive, so that those with it *are* worse off because they are found less attractive. Perhaps osmidrosis axillae *is* a pathological condition similar to naevus flammius (port wine stain), which harms the individual by making him less attractive. But other examples of putative diseases that do not harm can be found. In 1856 T.B. Curling considered that the frequent emission of sperm gave rise to 'constitutional symptoms of a serious character', and constituted the disease of 'spermatorrhoea' (Curling, 1856, p.386)! However, frequent ejaculation is not harmful, and so there is no such disease.

Other putative diseases are not diseases because even though they might result in the individual being harmed, they only harm the individual via undesirable human traits like prejudice. For example, Benjamin Rush thought that the black skin of Negroes was a disease which he called 'Negritude'. While it is true that one is worse off in a white racist society with black skin, and that one

208

would be better off white, we do not want to be the sort of beings where the mere possession of black skin counts as a disease (because of our prejudice). We are even better off not being prejudiced – if anything is the disease, the prejudice is! And so the disease of negritude does not exist.

Some putative diseases are not diseases because the nature of the condition is not as was supposed. For example, nephroptosis or floating kidney does not exist because there is no harmful condition with a nature consisting of a mobile kidney. The conditions mistaken as instances of floating kidney may do the individual harm – cases of renal colic were described as instances of floating kidney, and renal colic is harmful. But floating kidney does not exist because these conditions do not have the postulated nature of a mobile kidney. There is another more important reason why nephroptosis does not exist, and that is because such conditions do not constitute a natural kind.

Then there are cases where the disease does not exist because the conditions taken to be instances of that disease do not share an explanatory nature. For example, Richard Bright described a condition characterized by proteinuria, dropsy, and morbid changes in the kidney. However, it was soon realized that there were a number of distinct disease entities not sharing a common explanatory nature that resulted in such a clinical presentation. For example, essential hypertension and acute glomerulonephritis can produce this clinical picture, and there is no common (general) nature that they share. Hence Bright's disease does not exist.

In some cases a disease entity is taken not to exist not because the patients with it do not have a (specific) explanatory nature in common, but because the (higher-order) natural kind that they do fall into is not accorded the status of a disease-entity. For example, patients with diabetes mellitus fall into a number of distinct natural kinds, but because they share a (more general) explanatory nature, they constitute a (higher-order) natural kind. However, this natural kind is not accorded the status of a disease entity – it is what I have called a disease genus. The ascription of this status rather than that of a disease entity may be expressed as the conclusion that the disease entity of diabetes mellitus does not exist.

Similarly, it is sometimes claimed that certain conditions are not disease entities because they are merely forms of already recognized diseases. For example, Korsakoff's psychosis and Wernicke's encephalopathy are not distinct disease entities because they are merely forms of an already recognized disease – beriberi. When it was discovered that they shared the same pathology, it was concluded that such disease entities did not exist – only forms of an identical disease (beriberi) did (Malamud and Skillikorn, 1956, p.595).

Some diseases are not taken to exist because it has been discovered that individuals with the condition are merely at the extremes of the normal population, and therefore do not constitute a natural kind. For example, some have argued that Gilbert's disease does not exist because there is no natural boundary between those with Gilbert's disease and the normal population. However, I have argued that this does not show that the condition is not a disease – there may be many diseases, like essential hypertension, which are only deviations in degree from the norm. Gilbert's disease does not exist for another reason – it does the individual no harm.

Then there are conditions that may produce suffering, but which are nevertheless not diseases because they are the product of normal processes rather than some abnormal (disease) process. For example, towards the end of the nineteenth century it was widely held that (ordinary) menstruation was a pathological condition (Bullough and Voght, 1973, p.67). While it is true that women would be better off if they did not menstruate, we regard the process as a normal one, and hence the disease of menstruation does not exist. Similarly, the attempts of slaves to run away were not the product of the disease process of drapetomania, but the product of the normal processes of desire and belief formation. Hence drapetomania does not exist.

Some conditions are not taken to be disease entities because they are not processes. For example, the disease of club foot does not exist because club foot is a static defect, and not a process. This does not mean that it is not a pathological condition, for pathological conditions include static defects as well as processes. So in claiming that such diseases do not exist, we are not claiming that such pathological conditions do not exist.

Other conditions are not taken to be disease-entities because they are given the status of *signs* of a disease rather than that of a disease. For example, the disease of fever does not exist. This is not because one is not worse off being feverish, for one certainly is. It is not because patients with fever do not constitute a (higher-order) natural kind, because they do. But it is because it is taken to be a sign of a disease, and not a disease itself. It is seen as something that requires explanation, rather than a process that itself does the explaining.

Finally, some harmful processes, like starvation and drowning, are not regarded as diseases because they have obvious explanations, and have been for this reason classified differently in the past. We have come now to inherit this division, and so we do not consider that there is a disease entity of starvation.

## Conclusions

We started with two questions. Do we invent diseases or do we discover them? And do disease judgments express value-judgments or are they purely descriptive judgments? We are now in a position to give definite answers to these questions.

The concept of disease is a normative or evaluative concept. Judging that some condition is a disease is to judge that the person with that condition is less able to lead a good or worthwhile life. And since this latter judgment is a normative one, to judge that some condition is a disease is to make a normative judgment.

This then settles the Naturalist–Normativist debate. It is because the concept of disease is normative that we judge that conditions causing mental retardation and not genius are diseases. This normative view of the concept of disease explains why cultures holding different values disagree over what are diseases.

But does this mean we have to swallow Relativism? Does this mean that we cannot criticize Russian psychiatry for classifying behaviour they do not approve of (political dissidence) as due to a disease? Is political dissidence a disease-for-the-Russians but not a disease-for-us? Is there no absolute frame of reference in terms of which political dissidence is absolutely either a disease or not?

Normativism does not commit us to Relativism. When I judge that Hitler is an evil man, I am making a value-judgment. However, I do not commit myself to the view that Hitler is an evil-man-for-me, but not an evil-man-for-the-Nazis. This would be to judge that I am both against Hitler and for him in the same breath, and this is incoherent. Once I have judged that Hitler is an evil man, I judge that those who disagree are wrong, and set myself against them. So if I accept that disease judgments are normative, this does not mean that I have to accept that any condition is only a disease-for-me.

We have also seen that we do not discover what conditions are

211

diseases. That is, we do not discover disease status. Diseases are not diseases because they have a certain type of explanatory nature. We cannot discover whether some condition is a disease by discovering its nature because diseases do not constitute a higher-order natural kind in virtue of their sharing an explanatory nature.

Whether some condition is a disease depends on where we choose to draw the line of normality, and this is not a line that we can discover. Hence we cannot discover disease status. Rather, we invent disease status by imposing our distinction between disease and normality on the world.

But there is some truth to the view that our classifications can be correct (or false). There are some natural divisions among conditions that can be mirrored by our nosologies. Disease identity can be discovered, and not simply invented. Diseases can only be identical if they share the same explanatory nature, and diseases not sharing the same nature are different. And hence we can discover disease identity.

All this means that there is no easy solution to the classificatory problems with which I started. To judge that homosexuality is a disease, we have to first make a value-judgment. We have first to judge that we would be worse off if we were homosexual. If we have judged that we are worse off being homosexual, we have still to discover what process produces homosexuality before we can conclude that it is a disease. If homosexuality is the result of the normal processes of learning, then it will not be a disease. On the other hand, if it is the product of some abnormal (hormonal) process, then it can qualify as a disease.

Similarly, to decide whether smoking is a disease, we have to first judge that smoking is harmful. Having judged this, we have to discover what sort of process leads to the acquisition of the destructive pattern of behaviour. If it is a matter of simple habit formation (that is, a normal process), then we cannot conclude that smoking is a disease. On the other hand, if some abnormal neurological process, for example, the formation of a physiological addiction, is responsible for the behaviour, then the pattern of behaviour can qualify as a disease. Note that we might not come to call the habit of smoking a disease because, like barbiturate overdose, the condition does not have an obscure explanation. We might simply classify the condition as pathological.

Finally, hyperactivity will be a disease if we judge that the condition causing it is not just a nuisance to adults, but also harmful to the children themselves. In addition, if the process producing the behaviour is abnormal, like the overproduction of certain neurotransmitters, then the claim that hyperactivity is a disease will be strengthened.

In spite of the fact that there is no easy solution to the classificatory problems with which we started, this does not mean that there is a *carte blanche* to call anything we do not like 'pathological'. Even if we are not able to show that Russian psychiatrists have made a factual mistake in classifying political dissidence as a disease, we can still defend our values. Admitting that 'Hitler is an evil man' is only a value judgment does not mean that we cannot defend our values against others. It is because we value the states that we do that we become committed physicians working towards ridding man of certain conditions.

Does the fact that there is no easy solution to our classifactory dilemmas mean that the philosopher has no role to play in these debates after all? The answer is no. We need a philosopher to tell us that it is a mistake to make the Essentialist Fallacy, and go looking for a nature or essence which makes any condition a disease. Had this not been pointed out, we would still be searching for some special fact that would clinch the issue. Alas, there is no such fact.

But most importantly, the philosopher has provided an account of our concept of disease that will enable such debates to be settled. That such a definition still requires us to make a value-judgment does not mean that the philosopher has not helped. It just means that disease judgments, like moral judgments, are not factual ones.

# BIBLIOGRAPHY

Achinstein, P. (1977), 'Function statements', *Philosophy of Science*, vol. 44. pp. 341–67.

Ackerknecht, E. (1982), *Short History of Medicine*, Baltimore, John Hopkins University Press.

Acton, W. (1857), *Functions and Disorders of the Reproductive Organs*, John Churchill, London.

Agrios, G. (1978), *Plant Pathology*, New York, Academic Press.

Alexander, P. (1973), 'Normality', *Philosophy*, pp. 137–51.

Alzheimer, A. (1977), 'On a peculiar disease of the cerebral cortex', in D. A. Rottenberg and F. H. Hochberg (eds), *Neurological Classics in Modern Translation*, New York, Hafner Press, pp. 41–3.

Bailey, A. and Robinson, D. (1977), 'Does Gilbert's disease exist?', *Lancet*, vol. 1. pp. 931–3.

Baltozzo, G. *et al.* (1978), 'Evidence for a primary autoimmune type of diabetes mellitus', *British Medical Journal*, vol. 2, pp. 1253–8.

Barash, D. (1981), *Sociobiology: The Whisperings Within*, Glasgow, Fontana.

Barry, B. (1965), *Political Argument*, London, Routledge & Kegan Paul.

Batten, M. (1980), 'Earth's odd couples', *Science Digest*, pp. 60–76.

Benn, S. (1960), 'Interests in politics', *Proceedings of the Aristotelian Society*, vol. 60, pp. 121–140.

Bennett, J. (1976), *Linguistic Behaviour*, Cambridge University Press.

Bergler, E. (1956), *Homosexuality: Disease or Way of Life?* New York, Hill & Wang.

Bieber, I. *et al.* (1962), *Homosexuality: A Psychoanalytical Study*, New York, Random House.

Blackburn, S. (1971), 'Moral realism', in J. Casey (ed.) *Morality of Science*, vol. 44, pp. 542–73.

Boorse, C. (1975), 'On the distinction between disease and illness', *Philosophy and Public Affairs*, vol. 5, pp. 49–68.

Boorse, C. (1976a), 'Wright on functions', *Philosophical Review*, vol. 85, pp. 70–86.

Boorse, C. (1976b), 'What a theory of mental health should be', *Journal for the Theory of Social Behaviour*, vol. 6, pp. 61–84.

Boorse, C. (1977), 'Health as a Theoretical concept', *Philosophy of Science*, vol. 44, pp. 542–73.

Boyd, R. (1980), 'Materialism without reductionism: what physicalism does not entail', in N. Block (ed.), *Readings in Philosophy of Psychology*, vol. 1, London, Methuen, pp. 67–106.

Brandt, R. (1979), *A Theory of the Good and the Right*, Oxford, Clarendon Press.

Brown, R. (1977), 'Physical illness and mental health', *Philosophy and Public Affairs*, vol. 7. pp. 17–38.

Bucknill, J. and Tuke, D (1874), *A Manual of Psychological Medicine*, London, Macmillan.

Bullough, V. and Voght, M. (1973), 'Women, menstruation and nineteenth century medicine', *Bulletin of the History of Medicine*, vol. 47, pp. 66–82.

Bullough, V. (1979), *Homosexuality: A History*, London, Garland Press.

Callahan, D. (1973), 'The WHO definition of health', *Hastings Centre Studies*, vol. 1, pp. 77–88.

Campbell, E., Scadding, J. and Roberts, R. (1979), 'The concept of disease', *British Medical Journal*, vol. 2, pp. 757–62.

Canfield, J. (1963), 'Teleological explanations in biology', *British Journal of Philosophy of Science*, vol. 14, pp. 285–95.

Cartwright, S. (1851), 'Report on the diseases and physical peculiarities of the negro race', *New Orleans Medical and Surgical Journal*, vol. 7, pp. 707–9.

Charnov, E. and Krebs, J. (1975), 'Evolution of alarm calls: altruism or manipulation?', *American Naturalist*, vol. 109, pp. 107–12.

Clare, A. (1976), *Psychiatry in Dissent*, London, Tavistock Publications.

Clare, A. (1981), 'The threat to political dissidents in Kennedy's approach to mental illness', *Journal of Medical Ethics*, vol. 7, pp. 194–6.

Clinical Society of London, (1888), *Report of Myxoedema*, London, Longmans, Green & Co.

Cohen, G. (1978), *Karl Marx's Theory of History: A Defence*, Oxford Clarendon Press.

Cohen, H. (1961), 'The evolution of the concept of disease', in B. Lush (ed.), *Concepts of Medicine*, London, Pergamon Press.

Coiffi, F. (1982), 'Honours for craziness', *London Review of Books*, vol. 4, pp. 10–11.

Comfort, A (1967), *The Anxiety Makers*, London, Thomas Nelson.

Conrad, P. and Schneider, J. (1980), *Deviance and Medicalization*, London, C. V. Mosby Co.

Copeman, W. (1964), *A Short History of the Gout and the Rheumatic Diseases*, Berkeley, University of California Press.

Culver, C. and Gert, B. (1982), *Philosophy in Medicine*, Oxford University Press.

Curling, T. (1856), *A Practical Treatise on the Diseases of the Testis*, London, John Churchill.

Daniels, N. (1981), 'Health care needs and distributive justice', *Philosophy and Public Affairs*, vol. 10, pp. 146–79.

Davison, G. (1976), 'Homosexuality: the ethical challenge', *Journal of Consulting and Clinical Psychology*, vol. 44, pp. 157–62.

Davison, G. and Neale, J. (1978), *Abnormal Psychology: An Experimental Clinical Approach*, New York, John Wiley.

215

Dawkins, M. (1980), *Animal Suffering*, London, Chapman & Hall.

Dawkins, R. (1976), *The Selfish Gene*, Oxford University Press.

Downie, R. and Telfer, E. (1980), *Caring and Curing*, London, Methuen.

Dubos, R. (1959), *Mirage of Health*, New York, Harper & Row.

Dubos, R. (1965), *Man Adapting*, London, Yale University Press.

Dubos, R. (1968), *Man, Medicine and Environment*, London, Pall Mall Press.

Dupré, J. (1981), 'Natural kinds and biological taxa', *Philosophical Review*, vol. 90. pp. 66–90.

Enc, B. (1976), 'Reference of theoretical terms', *Nous*, vol. 10, pp. 261–81.

Engel, G. (1961), 'Is grief a disease?' *Psychosomatic Medicine*, vol. 23, pp. 15–27.

Engelhardt, T. (1974a), 'The disease of masturbation: values and the concepts of disease', *Bulletin of the History of Medicine*, vol. 48, pp. 234–48.

Engelhardt, T. (1974b), 'Explanatory models in medicine: facts, theories and values', *Texas Reports on Biology and Medicine*, vol. 32, pp. 225–39.

Engelhardt, T. (1975), 'The concepts of health and disease', in T. Engelhardt and S. Spicker (eds), *Evaluation and Explanation in the Biomedical Sciences*, Dordrecht, Reidel.

Engelhardt, T. (1976), 'Ideology and Etiology', *Journal of Medicine and Philosophy*, vol. 1, pp. 256–68.

Everitt, B. (1980), *Cluster Analysis*, New York, Halsted Press.

Eyer, A. (1894), 'Clitoridectomy for the cure of certain cases of masturbation in young girls', *International Medical Magazine*, pp. 259–62.

Faber, K. (1923), *Nosography in Modern Internal Medicine*, Oxford University Press.

Fales, E. (1979), 'Relative essentialism', *British Journal for the Philosophy of Science*, vol. 30, pp. 349–70.

Fales, E. (1982), 'Natural kinds and freaks of nature', *Philosophy of Science*, vol. 49, pp. 67–90.

Feinberg, J. (1984), *Harm to Others*, Oxford University Press.

Feldman, M. and MacCulloch, M. (1971), *Homosexual Behaviour: Therapy and Assessment*, Oxford, Pergamon Press.

Flegel, K. (1974), 'Changing concepts of the nosology of gonorrhoea and syphilis', *Bulletin of the History of Medicine*, pp. 571–88.

Flew, A. (1973), *Crime or Disease?*, London, Macmillan.

Flew, A. (1983), 'Mental health, mental disease, mental illness: the medical model', in P. Bean (ed.), *Mental Illness: Changes and Trends*, New York, John Wiley.

Foot, P. (1978), *Virtues and Vices*, Oxford, Basil Blackwell.

Foucault, M. (1965), *Madness and Civilization*, London, Tavistock Publications.

Foucault, M. (1973), *The Birth of the Clinic*, London, Tavistock Publications.

Frey, R. (1980), *Interests and Rights*, Oxford, Clarendon Press.

Garrett, S. (1970), *Pathogenic Root-infecting Fungi*, Cambridge University Press.

Geach, P. (1957), *Mental Acts*, London, Routledge & Kegan Paul.

Glover, J. (1970), *Responsibility*, London, Routledge & Kegan Paul.

Glover, J. (1977), *Causing Death and Saving Lives*, Harmondsworth, Penguin.

Glover, J. (1984), *What Sort of People Should There Be?*, Harmondsworth, Penguin.

Goosens, W. (1977), 'Underlying trait terms', in S. Schwartz (ed.) *Naming, Necessity, and Natural Kinds*, London, Cornell University Press, pp. 133–54.

Goosens, W. (1980), 'Values, health and medicine, *Philosophy of Science*, vol. 47, pp. 100–15.

Gould, S. (1977), *Ever Since Darwin*, Harmondsworth, Penguin.

Gould, S. (1980), *The Panda's Thumb*, New York, W. W. Norton & Co.

Gould, S. (1983), *Hen's Teeth and Horses' Toes*, New York, W. W. Norton & Co.

Gowers, W. (1904), 'Lumbago: its lessons and analogues', *British Medical Journal*, vol. 1. pp. 117–21.

Gull, W. (1873), 'On a cretinoid state supervening in adult life in women', *Transactions of the Clinical Society of London*, vol. 7, pp. 174–86.

Hamrin, B., Jonsson, N. and Landberg, T. (1964), 'Arteritis in polymyalgia rheumatica', *Lancet*, vol. 1, pp. 397–401.

Hare, R. (1972), 'Wrongness and harm', in R. Hare, *Essays on the Moral Concepts*, London, Macmillan, pp. 92–109.

Hare, R. (1979), 'What makes choices rational?', *Review of Metaphysics*, vol. 32, pp. 625–37.

Harré, R. and Madden, E. (1975), *Causal Powers*, Oxford, Basil Blackwell.

Harrison, M. and Bevan A. (1967), 'Early symptoms of temporal arteritis', *Lancet*, vol. 2. pp. 638–41.

Harsanyi, Z. and Hutton, R. (1983), *Genetic Prophecy*, London, Granada.

Hempel, C. (1965), *Aspects of Scientific Explanation*, New York, Free Press.

Henry, G. (1941), 'Organic mental disease', in G. Zilboorg (ed.), *A History of Medical Psychology*, New York, W. W. Norton & Co.

Hirschfield, M. (1936), *Encyclopaedia Sexualis*, New York, Dingwall-Rock.

Holt, A. (1936), *Diseases of Infancy and Childhood*, New York, Basic Books.

Horsfall, J. and Couling, E. (1978), *Plant Disease*, London, Academic Press.

Horton, B. and Magath, T. (1932), 'An undescribed form of arteritis of the temporal vessels', *Mayo Clinic Proceedings*, vol. 7, pp. 700–2.

Hubin, D. (1980), 'Prudential reasons', *Canadian Journal of Philosophy*, vol. 10, pp. 63–87.

Hun, T. and Prudden, P. (1888), 'Four cases of Myxoedema', *American Journal of Medical Science*, vol. 96, pp. 140–6.

217

Hunter, J. (1786), *A Treatise on the Venereal Disease*, London, John Churchill.

Huskisson, E., Dieppe, P. and Balme, H. (1977), 'Complicated polymyalgia', *British Medical Journal*, vol. 2, pp. 1459–65.

Illich, I. (1976), *Medical Nemesis*, Harmondsworth, Penguin.

Jakob, A. (1971), 'Concerning a unique disease of the central nervous system with noteworthy anatomical findings', *Archives of Neurology*, vol. 25, pp. 572–8.

Jellinek, E. (1952), 'Phases of Alcohol Addiction', *Quarterly Journal for the Studies of Alcoholism*, vol. 13, pp. 673–84.

Jobe, T. (1976), 'Medical theories of melancholia in the seventeenth and eighteenth centuries', *Clio Medica*, vol. 11, pp. 217–31.

Johnson, W. and Lyon, H. (1976), *Insects that Feed on Trees and Shrubs*, London, Cornell University Press.

Kardinal C. and Yarbro, J. (1979), 'A conceptual history of cancer', *Seminars in Oncology*, vol. 6, pp. 396–408.

Keen, H. (1981), 'The nature of the diabetes syndrome', *Medicine*, vol. 1, pp. 327–34.

Kennedy, I. (1983), *The Unmasking of Medicine*, London, Granada.

Kendell, R. (1975), *The Role of Diagnosis in Psychiatry*, Oxford, Blackwell Scientific Publications.

Kendell, R. (1976), 'The concept of disease', *British Journal of Psychiatry*, vol. 128, pp. 508–9.

Kendell, R. (1979), 'Alchoholism: a medical or a political problem?', *British Medical Journal*, vol. 1, pp. 367–71.

King, L. (1954), 'What is disease?', *Philosophy of Science*, vol. 12, pp. 193–203.

King, L. (1963), *The Growth of Medical Thought*, University of Chicago Press.

King, L. (1984), *Medical Thinking*, Princeton University Press.

Kinsey, A. (1953), *Sexual Behaviour in the Human Female*, Philadelphia, W. B. Saunders.

Kittrie, N. (1971), *The Right to be Different*, London, Johns Hopkins University Press.

Kraupl Taylor, F. (1979), *The Concepts of Illness, Disease and Morbus*, Cambridge University Press.

Kripke, S. (1980), *Naming and Necessity*, Oxford, Basil Blackwell.

Kugelberg, E. and Welander, L. (1956), 'Heredofamilial juvenile muscular atrophy simulating muscular dystrophy', *Archives of Neurology and Psychiatry*, vol. 15, pp. 500–8.

Lallemand, J. (1847), *A Treatise on Spermatorrhoea*, London, John Churchill.

Laufer, M. (1957), 'Hyperkinetic impulse disorder in children's behaviour problems', *Psychological Medicine*, vol. 19, pp. 38–49.

Lechewalier, H. and Solotorovsky, M. (1974), *Three Centuries of Microbiology*, New York, Dover.

Leplin, J. (1979), 'Reference and scientific realism', *Studies in the History and Philosophy of Science*, vol. 10, pp. 265–77.

Lewis, A. (1934), 'Melancholia: a historical review', *Journal of Mental*

*Science*, vol. 80, pp. 1–42.

Lewis, A. (1955), 'Health as a social concept', *British Journal of Sociology*, vol. 4, pp. 109–224.

Lewis, A. (1963), 'Medicine and the affections of the mind', *British Medical Journal*, vol. 2, pp. 1549–57.

Lewontin, R. (1982), *Human Diversity*, New York, H. Freeman & Co.

Linder, R. (1965), 'Diagnosis: description or prescription?', *Perceptual and Motor Skills*, vol. 20, pp. 1081–92.

Locke, J. (1965), *An Essay Concerning Human Understanding*, in J. W. Yolton (ed.), London, Everyman Library.

Long, E. (1928), *History of Pathology*, London, Ballière, Tindell & Cox.

Lugaresi, E., Gambetti, P. and Rossi, P. (1966), 'Chronic neurogenic muscular atrophies of infancy: their nosological relationships with Werdnig–Hoffman's disease', *Journal of Neurological Science*, vol. 3, pp. 399–407.

Mackie, J. (1976), *Problems from Locke*, Oxford, Clarendon Press.

Macklin, R. (1972), 'Mental health and mental illness: some problems of definition and concept formation', *Philosophy of Science*, vol. 39, pp. 341–65.

Malamud, N. and Skillicorn, S. (1956), 'Relationship between the Wernicke and Korsakoff Syndromes', *Archives of Neurology and Psychiatry*, vol. 76, pp. 585–96.

Mann, W. (1958), 'Bright's disease: the changing concept of a century', *Guys Hospital Reports*, p. 107, pp. 323–42.

Manning, A. (1979), *An Introduction to Animal Behaviour*, London, Edward Arnold.

Margolis, J. (1966), *Psychotherapy and Morality*, New York, Random House.

Margolis, J. (1969), 'Illness and medical values', *Philosophy Forum*, vol. 8, pp. 55–76.

Margolis, J. (1976), 'The concept of disease', *Journal of Medicine and Philosophy*, vol. 1, pp. 238–55.

Maudsley, H. (1867), *The Physiology and Pathology of Mind*, London, Macmillan.

Maudsley, H. (1868), 'Illustrations of a variety of insanity', *Journal of Mental Science*, vol. 14, p. 149.

Mayr, E. (1963), *Populations, Species, and Evolution*, London, Harvard University Press.

Mayr, E. (1976), *Evolution and the Diversity of Life*, London, Harvard University Press.

Meadows J., Marsden, C. and Harriman, D. (1968), 'Chronic spinal muscular atrophy in adults', *Journal of Neurological Science*, vol. 9, pp. 548–60.

Meddis, R. (1979), 'The evolution and function of sleep', in D. Oakley and Plotkin (eds), *Brain, Behaviour and Evolution*, London, Methuen, pp. 99–125.

Meiland, J. and Krausz, M. (eds) (1982), *Relativism: Cognitive and Moral*, Notre Dame, University of Notre Dame Press.

Mellor, D. (1977), 'Natural kinds', *British Journal of Philosophy of Science*, vol. 28, pp. 299–312.

Melzack, R. (1973), *The Puzzle of Pain*, Harmondsworth, Penguin.

Murphy, L. (1972), *History of Urology*, Springfield, Charles C. Thomas.

Nagel, E. (1979), *Teleology Revisited*, New York, Columbia University Press.

Nagel, T. (1979), *Mortal Questions*, Cambridge University Press.

Namba, J., Aberfeld D. and Grob, D. (1970), 'Chronic proximal spinal muscular atrophy', *Journal of Neurological Science*, vol. 11, pp. 401–15.

Newton-Smith, W. (1981), *The Rationality of Science*, London, Routledge & Kegan Paul.

Newton-Smith, W. (1982), 'Relativism and the possibility of interpretation', in M. Hollis and S. Lukes (eds), *Rationality and Relativism*, Oxford, Basil Blackwell, pp. 106–22.

Norris, F. (1969), 'Adult spinal motor neurone disease', in P. J. Vinken and G. M. Bruyn (eds), *Handbook of Neurology*, vol. 2, pp. 1–44.

Nozick, R. (1974), *Anarchy, State and Utopia*, Oxford University Press.

Offer, D. and Sabshin, M. (1966), *Normality*, New York, Basic Books.

Ord, W. (1878), 'On myxoedema, a term proposed to be applied to an essential condition in the cretinoid affection, occasionally observed in middle aged women', *Medical and Chirurgical Transactions*, vol. 61, pp. 57–78.

Parfit, D. (1984), *Reasons and Persons*, Oxford, Clarendon Press.

Patten, J. (1977), *Neurological Differential Diagnosis*, London, Harold Starke.

Petterssen, S. (1969), *Introduction to Meteorology*, New York, McGraw-Hill.

Pickering G. (1962), 'The nature of hypertension', *Lancet*, pp. 1296–304.

Platts, M. (1983), 'Explanatory kinds', *British Journal of Philosophy of Science*, vol. 34, pp. 133–46.

Potts, R. (1897), 'A case of masturbatory insanity', *Texas Medical Practitioner*, 2, pp. 7–9.

Preston, N. (1983), 'Is stuttering an illness?', *Journal of Paediatrics*, 41, pp. 135–6.

Putnam, H. (1976a), *Mathematics, Matter and Method: Philosophical Papers Volume 1*, Cambridge University Press.

Putnam, H. (1976b), *Mind, Language and Reality: Philosophical Papers Volume 2*, Cambridge University Press.

Putnam, H. (1983), *Realism and Reason: Philosophical Papers Volume 3*, Cambridge University Press.

Reynolds, M. (1983), 'The development of the concept of fibrositis', *Journal of the History of Medicine and Allied Sciences*, vol. 38, pp. 5–35.

Riker, A. (1939), 'Studies in infectious hairy root in nursery apple trees', *Journal of Agricultural Research*, vol. 41, pp. 507–46.

Rimoin, D. *et al.* (1969), 'Peripheral subresponsiveness to human growth hormone in the African pygmies', *New England Journal of Medicine*, vol. 281, pp. 1383–8.

Robertson, A. (1869), 'Notes on a visit to American Asylums', *Journal of Mental Science*, 17, pp. 19–26.

Ruse, M. (1971), 'Functional statements in biology', *Philosophy of Science*, vol. 38, pp. 87–95.

Ruse, M. (1973), *The Philosophy of Biology*, London, Hutchinson University Library.

Rush, B. (1785), *An Enquiry into the Effects of Ardent Spirits upon the Body and Mind*, New York.

Salmon, N. (1982), *Reference and Essence*, Princeton University Press.

Scadding, J. (1963), 'Meaning of diagnostic terms in broncho-pulmonary disease', *British Medical Journal*, vol. 2, pp. 1425–30.

Schrag, P. and Divoky, D. (1975), *The Myth of the Hyperactive Child*, Harmondsworth, Penguin.

Sedgwick, P. (1973), 'Illness – mental and otherwise', *Hastings Centre Studies*, vol. 1. pp. 19–40.

Sherman, P. (1977), 'Nepotism and the evolution of alarm calls', *Science*, vol. 197, pp. 1246–53.

Singer, P., Gould, S. and Luria, S. (1981), *A View of Life*, London, Bergamin Cummings.

Skultans, V. (1979), *English Madness*, London, Routledge & Kegan Paul.

Smythe, H. (1979), 'Fibrositis as a disorder of pain modulation', *Clinics in Rheumatic Diseases*, vol. 5, pp. 830–41.

Smythe, N. (1970), 'On the existence of pursuit invitation signals in mammals', *American Naturalist*, vol. 104, pp. 491–500.

Sorabji, R. (1964), 'Function', *Philosophical Quarterly*, vol. 14, pp. 289–302.

Spratling, E. (1895), 'Treatment for masturbatory insanity', *Medical Record*, 48, pp. 442–6.

Stockman, R. (1904), 'The causes, pathology, and treatment of chronic rheumatism', *Edinburgh Medical Journal*, vol. 15, pp. 107–16 and 223–35.

Sydenham, T. (1848), *Works*, in R. Latham (ed.), London, Sydenham Society.

Szasz, T. (1960), 'The myth of mental illness', *American Psychologist*, vol. 15, pp. 113–18.

Szasz, T. (1961), *The Myth of Mental Illness*, New York, Harper–Hoeber.

Szasz, T. (1972), 'Bad habits are not diseases', *The Lancet*, vol. 128, pp. 83–4.

Szasz, T. (1973a), *The Second Sin*, London, Routledge & Kegan Paul.

Szasz, T. (1973b), *Ideology and Insanity*, Harmondsworth, Penguin.

Szasz, T. (1976), *Schizophrenia*, Oxford University Press.

Temkin, O. (1971), *The Falling Sickness*, Baltimore, John Hopkins University Press.

Thomas, L. (1974), *Lives of a Cell*, New York, Bantam Books.

Thomas, L. (1979), *Medusa and the Snail*, New York, Bantam Books.

Thomas, J. (1966), 'Grue', *Journal of Philosophy*, vol. 63, pp. 289–309.

Toon, P. (1981), 'Defining disease – classification must be distinguished from evaluation', *Journal of Medical Ethics*, vol. 7, pp. 197–201.

Trotter, T. (1804), *Essay on Drunkenness*, Edinburgh, McLachlan & Stewart.

Uvarov, B. (1966), *Grasshoppers and Locusts*, Cambridge, University Press.

Veith, I. (1956), 'On hysteria and hypochondriacal afflictions', *Bulletin of the History of Medicine*, vol. 30, pp. 233–40.

Veith, I. (1965a), *Hysteria: The History of a Disease*, University of Chicago Press.

Veith, I. (1969), 'Historical reflections on the changing concepts of disease', *California Medicine*, vol. 110, pp. 501–6.

Victor, M., Adams, R. and Collins, G. (1971), *The Wernicke-Korsakoff Syndrome*, Philadelphia, F. A. Davis Co.

Werdnig, G. (1971), 'Two early infantile hereditary cases of progressive muscular atrophy simulating dystrophy, but on a neural basis', *Archives of Neurology*, vol. 25, pp. 276–9.

Whewell, W. (1840), *Philosophy of the Inductive Sciences*, London, Parker.

Whitbeck, C. (1976), 'The relevance of philosophy of medicine for the philosophy of science', F. Suppe and P. Asquith (eds), *Proceedings of the Science Association, Volume 2*, Ann Arbor: Edwards Brothers.

Whitbeck, C. (1977), 'Causation in medicine: the disease entity model', *Philosophy of Science*, vol. 44, pp. 619–37.

Whitbeck, C. (1978), 'Four basic concepts of medical science', in P. Asquith and I. Hacking (eds), *Proceedings of the Philosophy of Science Association Volume 1*, East Lansing, Philosophy of Science Association.

Whitbeck, C. (1981), 'What is diagnosis', *Metamedicine*, vol. 2, pp. 319–29.

Williams, B. (1973), *Problems of the Self*, Cambridge University Press.

Wing, J. (1978), *Reasoning about Madness*, Oxford University Press.

Winsor, E., Murphy, E., Thompson, M. and Reed, T. (1973), 'Genetics of childhood spinal muscular atrophies', *Journal of Medical Genetics*, vol. 197, pp. 143–56.

Woodfield, A. (1976), *Teleology*, Cambridge University Press.

Wootton, B. (1959), *Social Science and Social Pathology*, London, Allen & Unwin.

Wright, G. von (1963), *Varieties of Goodness*, London, Routledge & Kegan Paul.

Wright, L. (1968), 'The case against teleological reductionism', *British Journal for the Philosophy of Science*, vol. 19, pp. 211–23.

Wright, L. (1973), 'Functions', *Philosophical Review*, vol. 82, p. 139–68.

Wright, L. (1976), *Teleological Explanations*, Berkeley, University of California Press.

Zemach, E. (1976), 'Putnam's theory of the reference of substance terms', *Journal of Philosophy*, vol. 73, pp. 116–27.

# INDEX

223